SpringerBriefs in Public Health

SpringerBriefs in Public Health present concise summaries of cutting-edge research and practical applications from across the entire field of public health, with contributions from medicine, bioethics, health economics, public policy, biostatistics, and sociology.

The focus of the series is to highlight current topics in public health of interest to a global audience, including health care policy; social determinants of health; health issues in developing countries; new research methods; chronic and infectious disease epidemics; and innovative health interventions.

Featuring compact volumes of 50 to 125 pages, the series covers a range of content from professional to academic. Possible volumes in the series may consist of timely reports of state-of-the art analytical techniques, reports from the field, snapshots of hot and/or emerging topics, elaborated theses, literature reviews, and in-depth case studies. Both solicited and unsolicited manuscripts are considered for publication in this series.

Briefs are published as part of Springer's eBook collection, with millions of users worldwide. In addition, Briefs are available for individual print and electronic purchase.

Briefs are characterized by fast, global electronic dissemination, standard publishing contracts, easy-to-use manuscript preparation and formatting guidelines, and expedited production schedules. We aim for publication 8-12 weeks after acceptance.

More information about this series at http://www.springer.com/series/10138

Monica M. Taylor

Application of the Political Economy to Rural Health Disparities

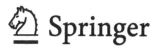 Springer

Monica M. Taylor
Colorado State University – Global Campus
Faculty-Healthcare Administration and Business
Greenwood Village, CO, USA

University of Maryland-University College
Adjunct Full Professor-Health Services Management
Adelphi, MD, USA

ISSN 2192-3698　　　　　　　ISSN 2192-3701　(electronic)
SpringerBriefs in Public Health
ISBN 978-3-319-73536-8　　　　ISBN 978-3-319-73537-5　(eBook)
https://doi.org/10.1007/978-3-319-73537-5

Library of Congress Control Number: 2018937341

Printed on acid-free paper

This Springer imprint is published by Springer Nature
The registered company is Springer International Publishing AG
The registered company address is: Gewerbestrasse 11, 6330 Cham, Switzerland

Preface

The life of this manuscript started with my concern for the downward trajectory in the health of the poor in a capitalistic society. While my emotion has not wavered over the past 10 years, I recently developed a growing concern for geographical poverty and the incomparable barriers that foster its subservience to capitalism. The legitimacy of this study is to correlate the unfortunate circumstances of rural populations with the interests of unpopular suspects, elitists. Their interests and influence places at risk, and at times, contradicts political opportunities to boost human and economic development for the rural poor in America.

Application of the Political Economy to Rural Health Disparities offers a unique analysis and perhaps a model to stimulate critical thinking on the plight of health disparities in rural populations. As Academics, we are driven to explore and develop solutions to the ever-growing problem of excess morbidity and premature mortality in disenfranchised communities. However, our research can become immersed with common rhetoric on causalities and endure re-emphasis on the problem with limited rhetoric for amenable resolutions. As a result, health disparities become static and in some cases, rather in some populations, worse.

As I write this book, I hope the viewpoints reflected in this manuscript dismantle the ideological philosophies that incite rural health disparities. I hope the evolving political climate pledges a compassion for public health endeavors, fiscal accountability and a commitment to improving life expectancy and quality of life for rural populations. I hope this further propagates civic and political engagement among rural constituents, and escalates a dialogue in the academic community that acknowledges the political and economic conditions that exacerbate rural health disparities.

Greenwood Village, CO, USA   Monica M. Taylor
Adelphi, MD, USA

Dedication

Dedicated to the most resilient children on earth, Christian, Chase, and Taylor; my loving mother; and my dearest friends, Tinequa and Anita, who believed in my dreams more than I did.

Psalms, 118:5

Introduction

This manuscript examines rural health disparities in the context of the political economy. This theory presumes there is a political and economic process that shapes public policy, which, in turn, influences the redistribution of public goods and impacts the built environment and behaviors in rural populations, rather unfavorably. This approach transcends conventional research on rural health. However, I found this lens rather necessary, especially because political theories appear nearly muted in the existing research on rural health disparities. Theories in the political economy offer a greater understanding of Government actions which inevitably create persistent geographical differences in health, which is salient at the national and global levels. This book hopes to stimulate further inquiries and research on the relationship between political theory and rural health disparities. Albeit, the relationship is quite simple and stated by Aristotle:

> "For as man is the best of all animals when he has reached his full development, so he is worst of all when divorced from law and justice." (p. 61)

And:

> "…the life which is best for men, both separately, as individuals, and in the mass, as states, is the life which has virtue sufficiently supported by material resources to facilitate participation in the actions that virtue calls for." (p. 393)

In both statements, Aristotle articulates an ideal state of well-being under the authority of a government with sufficient provisions for its citizens. The retrenchment of such provisions could then, according to Aristotle, compromise social engagement and the ability to achieve one's full potential. Therefore, I apply Aristotle's logic to the disparate conditions afflicting rural and extremely remote populations in America and feasibly demonstrate pathways in the political and economic process that facilitates retrenchment. The purpose of this book is to then expound the literary compass on rural health disparities and to juxtapose the pronounced effects of spatial differences and politics. This attempts a sharp deviation from the common juxtaposition of race and income, where income presents a more striking influence on health disparities (which is echoed profusely in the scientific literature). The point of convergence is the political economy as the central agent that triggers geographical differences in health. With this agenda at the forefront, the chapters are outlined accordingly: Chapter 1 provides a historical overview of the political economy perspective and its ontological variations (albeit progressive) from its theoretical underpinnings; Chap. 2 lends credence to prevailing economic factors that attenuate human development and advancement in rural populations; Chap. 3 illustrates the extent of social deviance in poor rural communities as the by-product of persistent economic instability; Chapter 4 applies economic development theories to the political agenda in the Trump Administration Chapter 5 concludes with further insight into the debilitating effects of the political and economic process on rural health outcomes.

Reference

Aristotle. (1992). *The politics* (Trans. T.A. Sinclair). London: Penguin. Page 61, 1253a, lines 32-4. Page 393, 1323b, lines 40-4. http://www.novelguide.com/aristotles-politics/top-ten-quotes

Contents

Chapter 1
Rural Health Disparities: The Political Economy

The atrocities in rural communities are unnerving, to say the least. The unrelenting issues of health disparities in life expectancy and morbid conditions, teenage pregnancies and scant options to secure critical social determinants requires sound theories followed by purposeful actions to bring stability and opportunities for advancement in rural areas.

At the heart of this book, is a proposal to apply political economy theory to direct the discourse on rural health disparities. My opinion is, that scientists have wasted time conjuring up sluggish interdisciplinary approaches that are underdeveloped and center on problems at the periphery (i.e. behaviors) rather than fundamental conventional politics. The political economy exposes the politics of government action or inaction to resolve the distressing social afflictions widespread in rural environments. This book argues that the political economy provides a rather illustrative compass of the systemic inefficiencies common in rural communities which affect physical and mental health and well being. The world-wide magnitude of the problem of rural health requires a solution that can meet its depth and breadth. This book intends to construe the prevailing discourse, theories, or interventions for rural health disparities as subordinate to the direction the political economy presents.

First, the word, 'economy' needs to be defined, explicitly, as it is characterized in the framework of the *political economy*. The *"economy"* in this context is concerned with economic events or economic affairs centered on capitalism. That is, capitalism in its accelerated form in the pursuit for profit absentia of government regulation (West 1969; Duffy 2015).

Capitalists would argue that this pursuit for profit inherently benefits the rest of society and will eventually increase the economic mobility of people in the lower socioeconomic stratum. However, the political economy tells us different (Sackrey et al. 2013). The political economy implicates capitalism as the source of class conflict. The political economy describes how such economic events affects other institutions, including political and social institutions. It theorizes capital accumulation as the great impetus in political decisions, ideologies or morale and further impacts

© The Author(s) 2018
M. M. Taylor, *Application of the Political Economy to Rural Health Disparities*,
SpringerBriefs in Public Health, https://doi.org/10.1007/978-3-319-73537-5_1

social institutions, rather negatively. Social, here, refers to society, its social development and availability of social goods to all populations and communities.

If we assess the origins of the political economy and how it was defined over time, early scientists such as Adam Smith and Karl Marx were renowned in this literature. Smith defined the political economy based on an economic philosophy and perceived it as a means to manage resources to generate wealth (Frey and Steiner 2012). Smith's account of the political economy undergirds classical economic rhetoric of market competition, the invisible hand, and challenges with economic liberalism. The early 1900s defined the political economy as the relationship between government and economic affairs (Okuonzi n.d.). Marx's philosophy progressed the dialogue from his predecessors and incorporated social and political dynamics in the context of economic affairs (Duffy 2015). Distinguished from his colleagues, economic theory was not described in isolation from such social and political dimensions. Marx's school of thought identified the economic order as a cause for constraint on social class structure and political institutions. He understood the relationship between class, profit maximization and any shift from investments in social infrastructure and labor to profits, could ultimately collapse the economic system sparking anti-capitalistic social movements against the current economic order (Humphrys and Collerson 2012). According to Duffy (2015), capitalism was responsible for class division and class struggle and therefore, exploitive. Alienation was inevitable under capitalism (more specifically, private property capitalist) as some individuals had access to luxury material resources while others lack this capability (West 1969). Labor divisions in the workplace caused worker degradation and little control over policies and conditions in the workplace.

For much of the historical discourse on the political economy, clear distinctions remained between the political and economical in terms of the actors who make decisions, their goals, and the institutions accountable for decision-making (Clark 2016). The actors in politics reflect decision-making by the collective with the intent to achieve justice and human rights. From an economic standpoint, consumers and producers make decisions to gain wealth and pursue market justice. The *institution* in politics consists of government where elections, campaigns and public policies are formulated. In economics, the *institution* is the marketplace where money and the exchange of goods and services occur. The concept of resource allocation is a shared theme within each dimension, albeit with different goals. The government distributes resources based on the needs of its citizens and the market system manipulates prices to encourage individual freedom to buy or sell products and services. While the distinctions in both disciplines are clear cut, to some degree, there is some overlap. Lawmakers advocate for policies that support the campaign contributions from wealthy (capitalist) donors and similar to governments, Corporations implement policies to control employee behaviors. In addition, the greater the degree of income inequality and wealth in corporations, the more power struggles and politics in the workplace. Hence, politics and economics demonstrate some level of interdependence, given the relevance of human interactions, methods to resolve conflict and goals for resource allocation within each discipline. At the same time, both disciplines show mutual exclusivity under these same circumstances.

Simply put, economic activities are directed by political decisions and economic stability drives government popularity (Frey and Steiner 2012). The government dictates economic activities through public policy formation. For example, the U.S. tax code can increase or remain unchanged based on the Administration in office (Republican or Democrat). In addition, policies are altered based on budget decisions, which include opportunities to increase or decrease investments in social welfare programs. Inflation and unemployment rates are guided by political decision-making. If economic policies demonstrate some level of success in boosting the economy, the public's response to the existing polity is acceptance, recognition and an opportunity for re-election.

Due to the interdependence and mutual interactions of both disciplines, various applications expound the topic of the political economy (Frey and Steiner 2012). Standard economics is one perspective and follows the expectation of government paternalism. The desire for government to expand provisions for social expenditures is assumed and public policies are oriented to reflect this ideology. However, real world circumstances, i.e. unemployment, limit the ability of governments to maximize or evenly distribute social benefits. The concept of public choice correlated with the political-economic interaction to reconcile the behaviors of politicians. Public choice also refers to voters and their biases in making decisions as well as their ability to make rational ones. Its derivative, social choice, reflects the challenge of self interests in politicians and bureaucrats when considering social welfare provisions. In addition, the econometric model reveals ways politicians constrain economic activities to ensure re-election by implementing economic policies that favor the populace.

The constitutional approach in political – economic interactions hinders on institutional conditions. Institutions make the rules which then dictate the political and economic process. Rule-making, structures and restricts behaviors and can influence human interactions. This approach reflects the modern political economy theory such that in the context of existing rules, institutions are perceived as endogenous, and therefore, any political or economic activities remain subjective. Public policies that serve institutional self-interests are regarded and economic decisions largely benefit the polity. This current school of thought differentiates from standard economic theory and its focus on welfare provisions.

Streeck (2011) considers the parameters that cause the capitalist version in the institutional political economy to function and specifies the problems governing capitalism. He describes institutional cynicism and the role of rule makers and rule takers in a capitalist order. People who make the rules permit certain actors, rule takers, to avoid rule compliance or the option to circumvent the rules in pursuit of their own self-interest. Streek describes differential endowments as inherent in the capitalist order. Capitalism does not evenly distribute resources across all classes. Individuals with the ability to pay for such resources, can enjoy them, in the absence of personal accountability to those who can not. The superior capitalist class or businesses have a greater advantage over the under-resourced classes. Non-capitalists may attempt to address government for a fairer share of resources, which rarely results in success. Relentless wealth is normalized under capitalism. Institutions don't impose limitations and therefore any motivation to maximize economically is considered rational and expected under capitalist order.

In the absence of regulation or political constraints on profit ceilings, inequality and social exclusion is inevitable (Streeck 2011). Consequently, the political agenda centers on restoration and redistributive efforts. Non-capitalists rely on the stability of an unrestrained economic system while elites remain unconcerned or unaffected by any forms of instability as accumulated riches provide them with long term financial security. Expanded wealth in free markets especially in technology and social relations propel the self interests of elites. Elites, then have the ability to adjust prices for goods and services with little regard, concern or reciprocity to non-capitalist. At the expense of other non-elites and potential solidarity, competition is maximized to enhance wealth, even if some are poorer as a result.

An exhaustive discussion on the varying (historical) assumptions of the political economy was a prerequisite to comfortably facilitate a greater understanding of this theory and how its concepts serve as the conduit for better literary discussions and effective policies on the elimination of rural health disparities. This chapter now turns from defining the political economy to ways this theory was applied to confront social issues. The remainder of this chapter expounds on the political economy of geography and the political economy of health due to their indisputable relevance to the conditions in rural areas and to further provide ontological reasons to address rural health disparities from a political economy perspective.

Political Economy of Geography

The political economy of geography offers meaningful dialogue to the discourse on rural health disparities. Capitalism and corporate decision-making is considered in investments in landscapes in certain areas. Regional economic developers can stimulate the economy in certain jurisdictions, i.e. rural, urban or suburban spaces, by encouraging entrepreneurship and offering incentives to attract large firms. Historically, regional economic changes occurred in certain spatial landscapes relative to others. According to MacKinnon et al. (2009), the motivation for economic geographical developments centered on capital accumulation. Corporate elites select areas for investments in land development and consideration of its effects on other socioeconomic groups remains a passive force. Class power and politics drive economic development decisions and this includes choices to close firms or expansions in international regions to remain profitable, notwithstanding its obligations to or consequences experienced by the weakened social class in urban or rural areas. Profit maximization and uneven development in non-profitable spaces is expected if political economic theory is applied to regional economic development.

Geographers developed interest in Marxian political economy as a result of the evolutionized global specification of capitalism (Wills 2000). With endorsements from multinationals, regional politicians and business, the emergence of global profit maximization came to fruition. The spatiality of capitalism intersected global borders, expanding its reach, technology and profits and transforming the discourse on political and economic geography worldwide. Laissez faire economics dominated global politics and accelerated capitalism was embedded in global social relations and decisions to participate in economic development in specified (urban) landscapes. The unequal development of landscapes at the transnational level prevailed at the consequence of local underdeveloped structures considered less profitable. Social exclusion remained pervasive at the global level, collective social commitments were minimized and labor relations were constrained.

Capitalism has geographical influence, worldwide, however rural regions, populations and the farming industry were particularly vulnerable to exploitation and market domination. The production, consumption (distribution) and accessibility of food is fundamental to a globalized political system dominated by Corporatism (Ehrenreich and Lyon 2011). Corporate elites are now interjected in multiple sectors of the food industry monopolizing food production in the U.S. and globally in international trade, crop production and retail, and therefore enhancing foreign competition in the agricultural market. The effects of this agri-business domination impacts small farmers and the rural poor. Farmers lack the capability to compete with agri-businesses in the free markets.

Multinationals have the resources to accelerate food production and this resulted in a degradation in food quality. Corporations used harmful pesticides and fertilizers on crops which compromised the health of farmworkers and consumers. Research studies showed that the quality of foods produced by Corporations (i.e. vegetables) demonstrated a reduction in minerals and nutrients compared to the crops that were once produced by rural farmers.

Corporate domination in rural spaces weakened quality of life and the availability of critical resources. The retrenchment of social benefits to farmers followed as institutions legitimized corporate behavior. Government subsidies to support farmers diminished. Farmers and the rural poor purchased food products at inflated prices. Farmers were converted to wage laborers. The rhetoric on the shortage of food supply was met with Corporate goals to increase food production without regard or acknowledgement of the consequences of free markets. Laissez faire economics in the agricultural industry brought an inequitable allocation of food supply which exacerbated food insecure environments, perpetuated poverty, especially among women (which consisted of 70% in the farming industry) and created an overall decline in health and well-being in thousands of farm workers who were hospitalized for pesticide related illnesses and injuries (General Accounting Office 2000). Ultimately, political will was minimized and what followed was inadequate global and national policies and provisions to mitigate food inequalities.

Geographers recognized that place and space, its production and reproduction, were critical to the wellbeing of the community that occupies it (Winterton et al. 2014). Spatial applications to measurements of well being aids in the identification of goals and objectives to build capacity, eliminate marginalization and sustainability and development efforts in rural locales. In rural areas, land development and environmental opportunities can either improve or hinder the well being of the people who live there. Local disadvantage, spatial inequalities and unsustainable infrastructure is the typical discourse in rural regions. Rural areas commonly lack social services and advancements in industry, and have been excluded from the benefits of the globalized production of space and landscape development. Rural populations were often subjected to the influence of multinationals and their domination in the agricultural industry. Changing the trajectory of the geographic scale necessitates consideration of macro-level influences and political dimensions.

Political Economy of Health

Reiterating concepts in the political economy, that is, the unequal distribution of resources and the politics of class power, permits its application to the realm of health disparities. Nowatzki (2012) describes a strong association between health, wealth and the political economy. In fact, Nowatzki asserts that health disparities have been underestimated given the lack of robust studies on the unequal distribution of resources associated with wealth. Wealth is commonly perceived as home and vehicle ownership, financial security and investments, however, extreme wealth and political power are concomitant. Measurements on wealth inequality and its links to health disparities require studies on macro-level income and political contributors such as median wealth per capita, income inequality, strength of union representation and policy variables linked to public expenditures on healthcare resources. Using these aforementioned variables in studies comparing wealth disparities in various countries, poorer population health, infant mortality and lower life expectancy was greater in countries with higher wealth inequality. Given these results, social policy resolutions should consider macro-level economic and political factors in the elimination of health disparities.

Health risk related behaviors can then be mediated (and explained) by the political economy of health framework (PEH) (Feldacker et al. 2011). The PEH vindicates personal choices and gives greater justification to political, economic and environmental inequities such as insufficient access to healthcare and income, class-power conflict, social exclusion, economic underdevelopment and limited mobility (Feldacker et al. 2011; Doyal 1995). These factors restrict individual (healthy) choices and facilitate risks for infectious and chronic diseases.

As we consider rural health disparities in the context of the political economy, scarce social determinants of health are ubiquitous in rural locations worldwide and these resources are critical to survival and impact quality healthcare delivery. For example, in Ghana, neonatal and maternal mortality are relatively high in this region (Masters et al. 2013). With neonatal mortality at 28% per 1000 live births and maternal mortality at 409 deaths per 100,000 women in 2008, 60% of rural women continue to have in home deliveries. Rural women in Ghana were aware of the benefits and reduced risk of complications for an in facility delivery, however, distance and mode and difficulty of transport to healthcare facilities was a primary deterrent to service utilization.

The HIV epidemic in Malawi disproportionately affects rural populations. Feldacker's et al. (2011) studies showed that distance to major roads and public health facilities and income inequality increased the likelihood of rural men and

Table 1.1 Concepts in political economy and its application to rural health disparities

Political	Economic
Resource allocation/class conflict resolution	Resource allocation/wealth accumulation
Social justice, humanitarian	Market justice
Resolution of social exclusion	Uneven land development
Public/social choice	Econometric model
Standard economics	Neoclassical economics
Marxism	Adam smith
Redistribution considerations	Capital accumulation
Solidarity	Competitive markets

women acquiring HIV. In the U.S., optimal stroke care in designated primary stroke centers is implausible in rural areas in the absence of technology feasibility and public policies that endorse e-health and telemedicine (Slade et al. 2012). A decade after China's transition to secure universal coverage for its population, significant progress, particularly among rural groups, was evident, however, rural residents continued to experience hardships in paying for healthcare services compared to their urban counterparts (Meng and Xu 2014). Vietnam experienced shortages in the distribution of physicians in its rural areas (Vujicic et al. 2011). Approximately 53% of physicians worked in urban areas, which consists of only 28% of the entire population. Urban wages were the primary catalyst to these concentrated employment rates in urban spaces.

These varying global examples show that the unequal distribution of the social determinants of health complicated opportunities for rural populations to obtain good health outcomes. Inadequate transportation, insufficient income, a limited supply of physicians to meet population demands, flawed insurance reform efforts and access to technology are clearly formidable investments that could alter the trajectory of rural health morbidity, mortality, injury and safety.

Justification: Political Economy and Rural Health Disparities

Table 1.1 summarizes the role of the two disciplines and serves to justify each concepts' theoretical relevance to the disparate health conditions in rural communities.

Table 1.1 affirms the political economy as a practical and credible theoretical stance to rural health. Of greater importance is the political willingness of governments to make provisions for equity in the distribution of the social determinants of health which could ultimately, equalize or lessen the burden of poor health in rural populations. The consideration of health as a basic right or as a commodity in free markets is challenged in some countries compared to others and provisions for universal care or fractioning of health care services, indeed falls under neoclassical philosophy driven by political decision-making.

References

Clark, B. (2016). *Political economy: A comparative approach* (3rd ed.). Praeger: Santa Barbara.

Crosby, R., Wendel, M., Vanderpool, R., & Case, B. (2012). Rural populations and health: determinants, disparities and solutions. New York: John Wiley & Sons.

Doyal, L. (1995). *What makes women sick: Gender and the political economy of health*. Rutgers University Press. New Brunswick, New Jersey.

Duffy, F. (2015). Marx's political economy. *Research starters: Sociology* (Online Edition).

Ehrenreich, N., & Lyon, B. (2011). *The global politics of food: A critical overview, 43 U*. Miami Inter-Am. L. Rev. Retrieved from: http://repository.law.miami.edu/umialr/vol43/iss1/3

Feldacker, C., Ennett, S., & Speizer, I. (2011). It's not just *who you are* but *where you live*: An exploration of community influences on individual HIV status in rural Malawi. *Social Science and Medicine, 72*(5), 717–725.

Frey, B., & Steiner, L. (2012). Political economy: Success or failure? *Contemporary Economics, 6*(3), 10–21.

General Accounting Office. (2000). *PESTICIDES improvements needed to ensure the safety of farmworkers and their children*. Retrieved from: http://www.gao.gov/new.items/rc00040.pdf

Hartley, D. (2004). Rural health disparities, population health, and rural culture. *American Journal of Public Health, 94*(10), 1675–1678.

Humphrys, E., & Collerson, J. (2012). Capital against capitalism: New research in marxist political economy. *Journal Of Australian Political Economy, 69*, 5–10.

MacKinnon, D., Cumbers, A., Pike, A., Birch, K., & McMaster, R. (2009). Evolution in economic geography: Institutions, political economy, and adaptation. *Economic Geography, 85*(2), 129–150. Retrieved from http://www.jstor.org/stable/40377292.

Masters, S., Burstein, R., Amofah, G., Abaogyec, P., Santosh, K., & Hanlon, M. (2013). Travel time to maternity care and its effect on utilization in rural Ghana: A multilevel analysis. *Social Science Medicine, 93*, 147–154.

Meng, Q., & Xu, K. (2014). Progress and challenges of the rural cooperative medical scheme in China. *Bulletin of World Health Organization, 92*, 447–451.

Nowatzki, N. (2012). Wealth inequality and health: A political economy perspective. *International Journal of Health Services, 42*(3), 403–424.

Okuonzi, S. A. (n.d.). *Political economy of health with reference to primary health care*. Retrieved from: https://tspace.library.utoronto.ca/bitstream/1807/6034/1/hp04008.pdf

Sackrey, C., Schneider, G., & Knoedler, J. (2013). *Introduction to the political economy* (7th ed.). Boston: Economics Affairs Bureau.

Slade, C., O'Toole, L., & Rho, E. (2012). State primary stroke center policies in the United States: Rural health issues. *Telemedicine & E-Health, 18*(3), 225–229.

Streeck, W. (2011). Taking capitalism seriously: Towards an institutionalist approach to contemporary political economy. *Socio-Economic Review, 9*, 137–167.

Vujicic, M., Shengelia, B., Alfano, M., & Thu, H. (2011). Physician shortages in rural Vietnam using a labor market approach to inform policy. *Social Science and Medicine, 73*(7), 970–977.

West, E. (1969). The political economy of alienation: Karl Marx and Adam Smith. *Oxford Economic Papers, 21*(1), new series, 1–23. Retrieved from http://www.jstor.org/stable/2662349

Wills, J. (2000). Political economy II: The politics and geography of capitalism. *Progress in Human Geography, 24*(4), 641–652.

Winterton, R., Chambers, A. H., Farmer, J., & Munoz, S. (2014). Considering the implications of place-based approaches for improving rural community wellbeing: The value of a relational lens. *Rural Society, 23*(3), 283–295.

Chapter 2
Rural Health Disparities: The Economic Argument

Economic instability and measures on wealth are common (and recent) indicators of population health. As race and ethnicity continued as a salient theme in the scientific literature associated with differences in disease prevalence and mortality, economic disparities and health disparities were increasingly more pronounced. Geographic differences, economic inequalities and health disparities have been substantiated in the discourse. This chapter explores the latter and shows the extent in which rural populations carried the burden of disease relative to their urban counterparts, in the context of various economic indicators. Relative to variables in the social determinants of health, this chapter evaluates the role of education, poverty, unemployment and income inequality on rural health outcomes.

Unemployment

During the recession (2007–2009), the unemployment rates for metropolitan areas peaked to 9.9% compared to rural areas, which rose at 10.3% by 2010 (United States Department of Agriculture 2017a, b, c). Since the recession, the labor market in nonmetropolitan areas have not fully recovered. There was nearly no growth overall in employment, job opportunities or labor force participation in those areas between the period of 2010 and 2013. After the recession (2011–2016), labor opportunities both accelerated and stalled in rural areas. While job opportunities have increased since 2014, rural areas still have not reached their employment levels from the pre-recession period. In contrast, labor market growth surpassed its pre-recession levels by 4.8% in metropolitan areas by the end of the second quarter in 2016.

Prior studies indicated that during periods of unemployment, mortality rates declined in the U.S. (Sameem and Sylwester 2017). This study drew comparisons between both rural and urban counties in the U.S. during three distinct recessions:

© The Author(s) 2018
M. M. Taylor, *Application of the Political Economy to Rural Health Disparities*,
SpringerBriefs in Public Health, https://doi.org/10.1007/978-3-319-73537-5_2

1990–1991, 2001 and 2007–2009. Rural counties demonstrated higher overall mortality rates during changes in the business cycle compared to urban populations. Regardless of gender, age or race (Black vs. White), mortality rates in rural populations exceeded death rates in urban populations. Of particular concern was the mortality rates for infants and children under the age of 5. In rural counties these rates more than doubled the rate for children in urban locales (Infant: 1969.8 and 826.8 and 428.2 and 193.3, respectively).

The major causes for mortality during fluctuations in the business cycle differed for both rural and urban counties. Heart disease was associated with changes in the availability of labor in urban counties. Studies showed links between stress and heart disease (CDC 2017a, b). When the economy prospered and the labor market was robust, people were worked harder, which elevated stress levels. Pollution was also linked to heart disease (Chen et al. 2005; Simoni et al. 2015). Urban counties were more exposed to pollution compared to rural populations, however, during periods of unemployment, this decreased exposure and the prevalence of heart disease in urban populations subsided.

External causes of death was associated with the business cycle in rural counties. External causes were fatalities from accidents in the workplace, home (fires), surgical mishaps, motor accidents, homicides and suicides. These fatalities were explained by the type of labor available in rural compared to urban counties. The number of fatalities decreased during recessions. Dependent on the business cycle, urban counties also experienced changes in mortality from vehicular accidents. This was closely associated with traffic and congestion found in urban locales during increased economic activity.

Studies also compared rural and urban population health status and the ability to utilize the healthcare system prior to the recession (2004–2007), post recession (2008–2009) and at the beginning of economic recovery (2010) (Towne et al. 2017). The recession period resulted in a loss of health care coverage. Employer-sponsored health insurance was the primary method for access to insurance in the U.S. With increased unemployment levels during the recession, the uninsured rose to nearly 50 million by 2010 (U.S. Department of Health and Human Services 2011). With gaps in coverage, fewer affordable options were available to the uninsured who sought healthcare. The options were more severe in rural areas, given the dearth in primary care and specialty care physicians (MacDowell et al. 2010).

During the pre and post recession period and the beginning of economic recovery, rural populations reported higher rates of disability compared to urban populations which further complicated the ability to access health care (Towne et al. 2017; Warren and Smalley 2014). Rural communities also reported less income and education. Rural populations were more unhealthy and refrained from seeking treatment during the entire timeframe of this study. Both populations reported good health outcomes prior to the recession than during the recession. Urban populations also abdicated healthcare, however, rural populations outpaced urban groups. The gap in seeking health care coverage among rural populations was likely due to a lack of health care infrastructure.

Education

Education attainment affects employment status. People with higher education had greater opportunities for employment, received higher wages and has less episodes of unemployment (U.S. Department of Agriculture 2017a, b, c). Overall, having college experience has been more favorable to job markets, particularly in urban areas. In rural areas, high school graduation rates have improved. Half of rural adults older than 25 lacked a high school diploma in 1970. By 2015, more than half of adults had a high school diploma or equivalent. Women in rural areas were more educated than men by 2015 and whites had higher education attainment compared to other racial and ethnic groups.

Urban and rural residents nearly converged on the number of adults without a high school diploma. However, a gap still remains between urban and rural populations in college completion rates, graduate and professional degrees. Between 2000 and 2015, college completion grew at a faster rate in urban populations. College attainment grew from 26% to 33% during this 15 year period. Rural areas experienced only a 4% increase (from 15% to 19%) during the same timeframe. Urban locales offered more job opportunities and favorable wages for college graduates compared to rural environments. Also, some rural residents may have attended college and chose to work in urban communities. These latter two factors could explain the lagged growth in college attainment in rural areas. Hence, poverty and inadequate education contributed to higher unemployment rates and greater poverty in adults and children who remained in rural communities.

Educational disadvantage had both direct and indirect effects on health (Probst et al. 2004). Limited education compromised the ability to seek healthcare (direct) as well as access to health insurance through employers (indirect). Studies suggested that racial and ethnic populations with limited education in rural locales suffered more severe health consequences. In Oregon, rural racial and ethnic populations with limited education reported more episodes of food insecurity (Gunter et al. 2017). Rural children were at greater risk of obesity as a result of specific family level indicators including low education attainment levels, poverty and access to affordable foods. Rural children with hearing loss were less likely to be diagnosed timely or to receive efficient pediatric care (Bush et al. 2017). Multiple barriers impeded care which included educational and socioeconomic status of the parents and a shortage in providers in rural areas.

Teen pregnancy rates in rural areas outpaced their urban counterparts (Ng and Kaye 2015). Rural teen pregnancy also exceeded their suburban counterparts. Rural teens were less likely to use contraception in their initial sexual experiences. By 2010, teen birth rates for children between the ages of 15 and 19, in rural counties, was one third higher than the U.S. average at 43 and 33 per 100,000, respectively. Rural counties demonstrated lower enrollment compared to urban counties. In South Carolina, rural counties had the highest teenage pregnancy rates compared to metropolitan areas in the state in 2013. In both cases, the most significant predictors of teen pregnancy included college enrollment, particularly in 18–24 year olds. More specifically, rural teens who did not enroll in college the previous year accounted for the 20% gap in pregnancy rates between their urban counterparts. Rural teens' perception of mobility is limited, given the prospects for economic advancement. In addition, a dearth in services and education contribute to higher rural teen birth rates.

Poverty

Nonmetropolitan areas, historically had higher poverty rates than urban areas (USDA 2017a, b, c). More specifically, poverty is higher in Southern states compared to other regions. Approximately 51% of the poor lived in the rural South. Growing gaps in poverty between metropolitan and nonmetropolitan areas became more prominent in the 1960s. In the 1980s, the average difference in the poverty rate in rural areas was 4.5% greater than urban areas. Rural areas experienced economic growth in the 1990s. By 2010, the gap was the smallest at 1.6%. However, since the recession, slowed economic recovery boosted the average poverty gap. In rural America, approximately 1.5 million children lived in poverty. The child poverty rate in rural areas consistently exceeded urban areas. Concentrated poverty increased in nonmetropolitan areas after the recession. The South experienced the highest poverty concentration relative to other regions in the U.S.. The poorest areas included the Mississippi Delta, Appalachia and Native American lands. By 2015, nonmetropolitan areas had a concentrated poverty rate of 7.7% compared to urban areas at 6.4%.

Scholarship on the interconnections between poverty and health disparities is both substantive and expansive. Income has been recognized for decades as a strong predictor for life expectancy. In the U.S., groups in the highest socioeconomic strata had a greater life span than populations in the lower economic stratum (Braveman et al. 2010). In rural areas, higher poverty rates attributed to the gap in mortality rates from potentially preventable diseases (CDC 2017a, b). Rural population experienced excess deaths from heart disease (25,000), cancer (19,000) and unintentional injuries (11,000). Behavioral risks factors in rural populations, such as smoking, obesity, limited physical activity, and lowered seat belt use transcend urban populations.

In the rural Mississippi Delta area, residents experienced persistent and concentrated poverty and racial discrimination (Kerstetter et al. 2014). Given their limited access to resources, residents consistently reported poor health. Infant mortality rates exceeded the state average. Residents in this region experienced higher overall mortality from all forms of cancer and heart disease compared to residents not housed in the Delta region (Gennuso et al. 2016). Although declining, these aforementioned mortality rates was still 20% higher than the rates in the U.S. and 10% higher in non-Delta regions. In addition, the Delta region faced the burden of sexually transmitted diseases, teen births, violent crime and single parent households compared to non-Delta regions.

By 2011, overall, individual level poverty in rural regions accounted for 133,000 deaths and 199,000 deaths occurred as a result of income inequality (Galea et al. 2011). Studies linked inadequate nutrition and food insecurity to concentrated poverty (Deller et al. 2015; Sadler et al. 2013). In North Carolina, rural populations were more susceptible to heat related illness and heat related deaths compared to urban populations (Kovach et al. 2015). In poor rural areas, agricultural work, noncitizenship and the number of mobile homes contributed to these health outcomes. In Illinois, more rural and the most urbanized counties had the highest monthly increases of hospitalizations caused by heat stress illness (Jaga et al. 2017). However, heat stressed illness and hospitalizations was the highest in remote sparsely populated rural areas. Cervical cancer incidence is greater among rural black women compared to urban blacks women (Singh 2012). The 5 year survival rates were at 50.8% and 60.2%, respectively. White women in nonmetropolitan regions also exceeded cervical cancer incidence rates of women in metro areas. While overall disparities in cervical cancer incidence declined in both populations, the gap in health outcomes remained salient.

Income Inequality

Income inequality, usually measured by the Gini index, Quantile Regression, Theil's entropy measure or the Atkinson index, refers to the distribution of income (The Brookings Institution 2017; De Maio 2007). The income inequality hypothesis (IIH) predicates differences in the distribution of income in a given area influenced individual health (De Maio 2014). The distribution of income matters when comparisons are made between the health of the top 10% earners and the middle and lower economic classes. The IIH claimed that health deteriorates with decreasing economic class. Researchers used the rationale in the IIH to explain and connect psychosocial, political economy, neoliberlism, and social trust research.

In the U.S., when income inequality levels increased, economic growth also increased in rural areas during this same time period and rural towns realized some population increases (USDA 2017a, b, c). The Obama Administration brought economic opportunities to rural areas. Job growth reduced unemployment rates and raised incomes for rural adults by nearly 6% in the past 2 years as a result of these efforts. However, legislative changes to increase the minimum wage presented a more directive approach to lessen income inequality and raise the incomes of the poor, overall, especially in rural areas.

Income inequality has come to the forefront of political agendas in the U.S. in recent years. The income gap widened and studies attributed growing income inequality to excessive poverty. In fact, studies implicated rising income inequality exacerbated rural child poverty (USDA 2017a, b, c). The rise in income inequality explained the 93% increase in rural child poverty between the years 2003–2014. Corak (2013) suggested that benefits in the human capital of children could raise their potential for economic mobility as adults. Corak's studies showed that countries with high income inequality levels, including the U.S., stagnated intergenerational mobility. In a global study, less earnings were available across generations in countries with high income inequality levels. A child's opportunities for economic mobility was hampered by family background, however depolarized labor markets and advancements in progressive public policies could reverse and equalize economic outcomes.

Many researchers, both nationally and globally, established a link between income inequality, wealth, health and mortality (Naoki et al. 2009; Pickett and Wilkinson 2015; Hajat et al. 2011). There has been an ongoing debate in the literature on the validity of the IIH. Zheng's (2012) studies found income inequality was detrimental to health, albeit the effects were only evident after 5 years. Zheng found the association between income inequality and mortality had an even more pronounced effect at 7 years and its influence decreased after 12 years. Studies in Africa found variations in mortality and income distribution evident in populations between the ages of 15–39 (Dorling et al. 2007). European studies did not support the effects of income inequality on health inequalities and attributed health differences to the association between education and health (Hoffmann et al. 2016). In the U.S. county level studies showed the association between income inequality and adverse mortality outcomes varied (Yang et al. 2012). In counties with death rates at 7.7 per 1000, income inequality had no effect. However, counties with death rates at 9.9 per 1,000, income inequality levels mattered. These findings were also confirmed for rural counties. In such counties, Yang et al. (2012) discovered that a one unit decrease in income inequality improved mortality rates.

Kragten and Rözer (2017) found high income inequality levels weakened social trust and caused psychosocial stress which ultimately compromised health. Differences in the flow of resources (income) resulted in competition and lead to stress and susceptibility to unhealthy behaviors. Other studies claimed increases in wealth, simultaneously reduced the risk of mortality. In a study conducted on 21,000 U.S. citizens, persons with assets greater than 500,000 had longer life expectancy. Comparably, U.S. citizens with deficient net worth had a 62% higher risk of mortality.

Health insurance programs, such as Medicaid and Employer Sponsored Health Insurance (ESHI), impacted income inequality levels (Kaestner and Lubotsky 2016). While rarely discussed in the discourse on income inequality, government benefits and individual health expenditures could enhance or compromise economic well being. The implementation of the Affordable Care Act not only reduced the number of uninsured, significantly but individuals in the lower economic strata benefitted the most. In kind income subsidies were available in the marketplace based on income eligibility criteria. The amount of the subsidies decreased with higher incomes (Centers for Medicare and Medicaid Services 2015). The ACA, therefore, added to the reduction in income inequality. Generally, persons in the lowest economic deciles received added income to offset the cost of insurance premiums, demonstrating that the poor profited the most from Medicaid expansion. On the contrary, Employer Sponsored Health Insurance widened income inequality as tax rates and premiums continued rise with income.

Conclusion

What is of central importance to rural health, and this chapter is the interrelationship of the IIH and political decisions to disinvest in public welfare and infrastructure Kawachi et al. (1997). In more equal economies, populations enjoy opportunities to access the social determinants and health and social services (Lynch et al. 1997). As described previously, government in-kind provisions to vulnerable groups builds their wealth.

Across all indicators described in this chapter, the IIH offers more context to the relationship between rural health disparities and the economic argument. If the IIH is true, then poverty is exacerbated by the inequitable distribution of income. The unfair distribution of income resulted in steeper poverty. If poverty alleviation is a meaningful and attainable goal in U.S. politics, then policies aimed to increase income, i.e. raising the minimum wage, would narrow the income gap between the rich and the poor.

Income distribution impacts the availability of social capital, including access to education and employment options. The political economy informs us that political decisions determine the extent in which the aforementioned benefits are evenly distributed throughout the population. Scant opportunities for economic stability, wealth, educational attainment and employment options is the prevailing discourse for dismal rural health outcomes. Health disparities in rural populations are exacerbated by geographical limitations in resources. In the absence of state investments towards prevention programs to improve reproductive care, college preparation, or healthcare services, at the very least, equitable to urban locales, health disparities in rural Americans will only worsen.

References

Braveman, P. A., Cubbin, C., Egerter, S., Williams, D. R., & Pamuk, E. (2010). Socioeconomic disparities in health in the United States: What the patterns tell us. *American Journal of Public Health, 100*(Suppl 1), S186–S196.

Bush, M., Kaufman, M., & McNulty, B. (2017). Disparities in access to pediatric hearing health care. *Current Opinion in Otolaryngology & Head and Neck Surgery, 25*(5), 359–364.

Centers for Disease Control and Prevention. (2017a). *Cardiovascular disease and occupational factors*. Retrieved from: https://www.cdc.gov/niosh/topics/heartdisease/default.html

Centers for Disease Control and Prevention. (2017b). *Rural Americans at higher risk of death from five leading causes*. Retrieved from: https://www.cdc.gov/media/releases/2017/p0112-rural-death-risk.html

Centers for Medicare and Medicaid Services. (2015). *"March 31, 2015 effectuated enrollment snapshot."* Fact sheet, June 2. https://www.cms.gov/Newsroom/MediaReleaseDatabase/Fact-sheets/2015-Fact-sheets-items/2015-06-02.html

Chen, L., Knutsen, S., Shavlik, D., Beeson, D., Peterson, F., Ghamsary, M., & Abbey, D. (2005). The association between fatal coronary heart disease and ambient particulate air pollution: Are females at greater risk? *Environmental Health Perspectives, 113*, 1723–1729.

Corak, M. (2013). Income inequality, equality of opportunity, and intergenerational mobility. *Journal of Economic Perspectives, 27*(3), 79–102.

De Maio, F. (2007). Income inequality measures. *Journal of Epidemiology and Community Health, 61*(10), 849–852.

De Maio, F. G. (2014). Income inequality hypothesis. In *The Wiley Blackwell encyclopedia of health, illness, behavior, and society*. (pp. 1223–1228). Chicester: John Wiley & Sons.

Deller, S., Canto, A., & Brown, L. (2015). Rural poverty, health and food access. *Regional Science Policy and Practice, 7*(2), 61–74. https://doi.org/10.1111/rsp3.12056.

Dorling, D., Mitchell, R., & Pearce, J. (2007). The global impact of income inequality on health by age: An observational study. *British Medical Journal, 335*, 873–875.

Galea, S., Tracy, M., Hoggatt, K., DiMaggio, C., & Karpati, A. (2011). Estimated deaths attributable to social factors in the United States. *American Journal of Public Health, 101*, 1456–1465.

Gennuso, K. P., Jovaag, A., Catlin, B. B., Rodock, M., & Park, H. (2016). Assessment of factors contributing to health outcomes in the eight states of the Mississippi Delta Region. *Preventing Chronic Disease, 13*, E33.

Gunter, K. B., Jackson, J., Tomayko, E. J., & John, D. H. (2017). Food insecurity and physical activity insecurity among rural Oregon families. *Preventive Medicine Reports, 8*, 38–41.

Hajat, A., Kaufman, S., Rose, K., Siddiqi, A., & Thomas, J. (2011). Long-term effects of wealth on mortality and self-rated health status. *American Journal of Epidemiology, 173*(2), 192–200.

Hoffmann, R., Yannan, H., de Gelder, R., Menvielle, G., Bopp, M., & Mackenbach, J. P. (2016). The impact of increasing income inequalities on educational inequalities in mortality – An analysis of six European countries. *International Journal for Equity in Health, 16*, 1–12.

Jaga, J. S., Grossman, E., Navon, L., Sambanis, A., & Dorevitch, S. (2017). Hospitalizations for heat-stress illness varies between rural and urban areas: An analysis of Illinois data, 1987–2014. *Environmental Health: A Global Access Science Source, 16*, 1–10.

Kaestner, R., & Lubotsky, D. (2016). Health insurance and income inequality. *Journal of Economic Perspectives, 30*(2), 53–78.

Kawachi, I., Kennedy, B. P., Lochner, K., Prothrow-Stith, D. (1997). Social capital, income inequality, and mortality. *American Journal of Public Health, 87*(9), 1491–1498.

Kerstetter, K., Green, J. J., & Phillips, M. (2014). Collective action to improve rural community wellbeing: Opportunities and constraints in the Mississippi Delta. *Rural Society, 23*(3), 257–269.

Kovach, M. M., Konrad, I. E., & Fuhrmann, C. M. (2015). Area-level risk factors for heat-related illness in rural and urban locations across North Carolina, USA. *Applied Geography, 60*, 175–183.

Kragten, N., & Rözer, J. (2017). The income inequality hypothesis revisited: Assessing the hypothesis using four methodological approaches. *Social Indicators Research, 131*, 1015. https://doi.org/10.1007/s11205-016-1283-8.

Lynch, J. W., Kaplan G. A., & Salonen, J. T. (1997). Why do poor people behave poorly? Variation in adult behaviors and pschosocial characteristics by stages of the socioeconomic lifecourse, *Social Science and Medicine, 44*(6), 809–819.

MacDowell, M., Glasser, M., Fitts, F., Nielsen, K., & Hunsaker, M. (2010). A national view of rural health workforce issues in the USA. *Rural and Remote Health, 10*(3), 1531.

Naoki, K., Grace, S., Ichiro, K., van Dam, R. M., Subramanian, S. V., & Zentaro, Y. (2009). Income inequality, mortality, and self rated health: Meta-analysis of multilevel studies. *BMJ: British Medical Journal, 7731*, 1178.

Ng, A. S., & Kaye, K. (2015). *Sex in the (Non)City: Teen childbearing in rural America*. Washington, DC: The National Campaign to Prevent Teen and Unplanned Pregnancy. Retrieved from: https://thenationalcampaign.org/sites/default/files/resource-primary-download/sex-in-the-non-city-final_0.pdf.

Pickett, K. E., & Wilkinson, R. G. (2015). Income inequality and health: A causal review. *Social Science Medicine, 128*, 316–326.

Probst, J. C., Moore, C. G., Glover, S. H., & Samuels, M. E. (2004). Person and place: The compounding effects of race/ethnicity and rurality on health. *American Journal of Public Health, 94*(10), 1695–1703.

Sadler, R. C., Gilliland, J. A., & Arku, G. (2013). Community development and the influence of new food retail sources on the price and availability of nutritious food. *Journal of Urban Affairs, 35*, 471–491.

Sameem, S., & Sylwester, K. (2017). The business cycle and mortality: Urban versus rural counties. *Social Science & Medicine, 175*, 28–35.

Simoni, M., Baldacci, S., Maio, S., Cerrai, S., Sarno, G., & Viegi, G. (2015). Adverse effects of outdoor air pollution in the elderly. *Journal of Thoracic Disease, 7*, 34–45.

Singh, G. (2012). Rural-urban trends and patterns in cervical cancer mortality, incidence, stage, and survival in the United States, 1950-2008. *Journal of Community Health, 37*(1), 217–223.

The Brookings Institution. (2017). *Stretchy ends: The shape of income inequality*. Retrieved from: https://www.brookings.edu/research/stretchy-ends-the-shape-of-income-inequality/

Towne, P., Hardin, B., & Glover. (2017). Health & access to care among working-age lower income adults in the great recession: Disparities across race and ethnicity and geospatial factors. *Social Science & Medicine, 182*, 30–44.

U.S. Department of Agriculture. Economic Research Service. (2017a). Rural employment and unemployment. Retrieved from: https://www.ers.usda.gov/topics/rural-economy-population/employment-education/rural-employment-and-unemployment/

U.S. Department of Agriculture. Economic Research Service (2017b). *Rural education at a glance, 2017 Edition*. Retrieved from: https://www.ers.usda.gov/webdocs/publications/83078/eib-171.pdf?v=42830

U.S. Department of Agriculture. Economic Research Service. (2017c). *Poverty overview: Rural poverty and well-being*. Retrieved from: https://www.ers.usda.gov/topics/rural-economy-population/rural-poverty-well-being/poverty-overview/

U.S. Department of Health and Human Services. (2011). *Overview of the uninsured in the United States: A summary of the 2011 current population survey*. Retrieved from: https://aspe.hhs.gov/basic-report/overview-uninsured-united-states-summary-2011-current-population-survey

Warren, J., & Smalley, K. (2014). *Diabetes in rural areas. Rural public health: Best practices and preventive models*. New York: Springer Publishing Company.

Yang, T., Chen, V. Y., Shoff, C., & Matthews, S. A. (2012). Using quantile regression to examine the effects of inequality across the mortality distribution in the U.S. counties. *Social Science & Medicine, 74*, 1900–1910.

Zheng, H. (2012). Do people die from income inequality of a decade ago? *Social Science & Medicine, 75*, 36–45.

Chapter 3
Social Disorganization in Rural Communities

The Rural Mystique is a social construct and implies a built nostalgia or glorification is associated with one's image about rural environments (Brown and Schaft 2011). It is a contemporary mindset, albeit, uninformed, due to the social realities that exist in the current rural landscape. Hardly, does the concept of rurality achieve clear comparisons to its urban counterparts on measures of economic, demographic, environmental or social characteristics. Rather, the idyllic landscape of uniformity, social organization, cultural values and the perception of moral character for the people who live there feed this social construction of place.

The symbolic images of rural as an organic community is divergent from the realities of its contemporary social condition. As previously described, when political economy theory enters the discourse, manifestations and/or the extent of social problems and inequalities are associated with political decisions that govern the inadequate supply of or inequitable distribution of wealth and resources. This theory explains how politics shape social problems (Miller 1976). The rural landscape is not absent from the consequences of such political decisions. This chapter uses the concepts in the political economy to explain the breakdown of a social system portrayed through population depletion, violation in social norms, uncovers theories that predict rural crime patterns, health disparities and finally, how capitalism predetermines and profits from social disorder in rural locales.

Population Loss

Population density has been challenging in rural communities. Rural communities in America lack population growth. The net loss of out-migration exceeded in-migration (Reichert et al. 2014). With deficient economic resources, out-migration of high school graduates is expected. In migration to rural counties in the U.S. is less attractive to people in their twenties and thirties and consequently, is a greater

© The Author(s) 2018
M. M. Taylor, *Application of the Political Economy to Rural Health Disparities*,
SpringerBriefs in Public Health, https://doi.org/10.1007/978-3-319-73537-5_3

contributor to the decline in population growth. Insufficient access to urban areas further augmented population loss. Minimal luxuries, conveniences, dining options or areas of entertainment facilitated dwindling demographics. What is arguably more decisive are the factors that shape individual decisions to return to these vulnerable communities. Limited employment served as a primary cause for out-migration and was a barrier to return migration for people with advanced degrees. However, family bonds largely supported return migration. Raising a family and experiencing wage cuts was an acceptable trade-off. Safety, community cohesion and community familiarity stimulated preferences to move back. In addition, family owned businesses also motivated returning migrants.

Rural Crime and Social Disorganization Theory

Mainstream criminal theories were centered on social and economic conditions in urban geographical spaces. Contemporary scholarship applied such theories to rural areas and reconstructed how rurality was defined to epitomize the global forces that shape all communities.

Social Disorganization Theory (SDT) is used to explain the spatial distribution of crime patterns in certain areas (Harbeck 2015). Distinct from other crime theories, SDT explores the ecosocial context in which crime infestation persists rather than the individual who committed the crime. Residential instability, ethnic diversity, collapse in family structure, unemployment rates, poverty and population size are indicators commonly measured in SDT (Moore and Sween 2015). SDT attends to the capability of social institutions to maintain public order in some geographical spaces relative to others. According to SDT, declines in social order materialized as a result of failure from a range of social institutions including community organizations, businesses, law enforcement, health care, religious organizations, or community organizations. Neighborhoods with minimal criminal activity are endowed with a spectrum of collective resources, skills and determination to boost quality of life.

SDT derived in the early nineteenth century from Belgian sociologist, Adolphe Quetelet, who studied causes for crime rates primarily in urban areas (Gottfredson and Hirschi 1990). Quetelet attested to the long term stability of crime in communities and proclaimed that newly migrated groups or rare elements in the environment attributed to criminal activity. SDT evolutionized and researchers such as Thomas and Znaniecki (1996) added individual behaviors and belief systems due to a community acculturation process enhanced crime rates. With a focus still on urban spaces, Paul and Burgess (Soukhanov 2004; Gottfredson and Hirschi 1990) adapted the concept of ecology and predicated the direction of crime (minimal or excessive) as constructed by an exchange between human interaction and environmental resources and structures. Renowned as concentric zone theory, Paul and Burgess classified ecological spaces as zones and elucidated five favorable and disadvantaged zones omnipresent in urban areas: central business district, transitional, working class with tenement housing, residential which consisted of single family homes, and the suburban commuter zone. The transitional zone was considered the least desired with higher crime rates and represented an intense competition of resources, a point of entry for new migrants, cultural diversity, high unemployment rates, minimal educational attainment and low real estate values. Various researchers applied this theory to urban spaces in different countries and their findings substantiated Paul and Burgess' research.

Scholarship theories on rural crime was neglected and the assumption of uniformity, safety and social control prevailed (Weisheit et al. 2006). Theorists continued to make modifications to SDT, over decades, however, much of the discourse remained on its application to urban crime. The Chicago School added concepts of collective efficacy to study crime infestation in Chicago cities (Can 2014). Collective efficacy studies showed that social trust, cohesiveness and a neighbor's proclivity to reprimand (child) misconduct predicted a person's susceptibility to being victimized. In addition, social capital in urban cities was linked to youth crime. The presence of positive enforcement, role models and educational sponsors determined the extent of youth criminal activity and amenability to gang associations.

Clearly, there is a lag in the research literature on rural crime. Scholars primarily focused criminological theories to urban communities. In addition, criminality on a rural scale was often perceived as a diminutive construction of the urban crisis and finding consistent data measurements on rural indicators has been challenging (Kaylen and Pridemore 2013). However, developing scholarship emerged that explained the motivations for persons to commit crimes in rural areas differed from urban areas (Deller and Deller 2010). In urban areas, environmental transitions from residential to commercial property caused residents to live in substandard housing and communities, increased poverty and the collapsed the family structure consequently, increased stress and sparked juvenile delinquency rates (Shaw and McKay 1942). Residents were less likely to reprimand problematic behavior among youths. However, in rural areas, Kaylen and Pridemore (2013) found that a disruption in family structure which often prompted crime among youths.

Historically, the scientific literature has been divided on SDT's suitability to predetermine the extent of crimes in rural areas. Some researchers argued that the indicators for SDT was not a valid predictor on crime in rural communities (Kaylen and Pridemore 2013; Wells and Weisheit 2004). Moore et al. (2015) found that residential instability, ethnic diversity and female headed households were determinants for crimes among youths in 48 rural counties in the U.S. In fact, residential instability was a large predictor for specific criminal activities which included rape, robbery, assault and weapons possession. Moore's findings did not show that residential stability predicted the likelihood to commit murder. Ethnic diversity in rural counties demonstrated the greatest predictor for loss of social control in rural counties for all crimes in their analyses while family disruption only predicted robbery, assault, and weapons. Comparable to urban crime patterns, Moore's research found that poverty in rural areas only predicted the ability to commit murder. Living in poverty in rural counties did not predict any other crime indices and being unemployed did not impact juvenile crime rates as predicted in urban locales. In addition, rural counties that were adjacent to metropolitan areas did not demonstrate any spillover effects of juvenile delinquency.

Incarceration Rates: Rural-Urban Divide

The idyll nature of the rural landscape offers the impression that crime is not pervasive in these areas. This could not be further from reality. According to scientific evidence, poverty and uptake in criminal activity is inevitable. Historically, urban crime rates have been higher than in rural areas (Donnermeyer 2007). However, the rate of rural crime has increased dramatically since the 1960s (McGranahan 1986). In fact, by the 1970s rural crime rates exceeded metropolitan crime rates from the 1960s. Rural and big city urban crimes are increasing at the same rate. Property crimes were more prevalent from the 1960 to 1980s in rural locales and involved a high percentage of youths. Theft in farm crimes cost the industry millions (Jones 2012). Murder rates were high mainly in concentrated poverty-stricken rural areas (Lee and Ousey 2001). In the late 1990s–2000s, immigration regulations at the Mexican border caused an increase of low skilled Hispanic populations to rural areas (Shihadeh and Barranco 2010). Rural communities typically had employment demands for low skilled workers and rural employers favored migrating Hispanics given their satisfaction with lower wages. This tension, strained the availability for employment resources between the existing black population and predominantly non-white residents and contributed to the significant rise in crime rates, particularly, among non-Hispanic whites. In 2013, rural youths in the Lesbian, Gay, Bisexual, and Transgender population were 1.5 times as likely to experience physical assault compared to their urban and suburban counterparts (The National Center for Victims on Crime 2017). Overall, the chances of victimization among youths between the ages of 15–17 years was 3.9 times greater than their urban counterparts and 4 times higher than suburban youths in the same age group.

The geography of the prison population has changed significantly (Kang-Brown and Subramanian 2017). Typically, urban residents populated U.S. jails. Trends in incarceration rates showed that urban crime declined in America's cities as rural criminal actively rose sharply. Currently, prisoners in U.S. jails were primarily from small rural counties. Incarceration rates among rural women outpaced their urban counterparts. In fact, white rural women from small rural counties contributed to the surge in incarceration rates. Concurrently, in urban counties, black and white incarceration rates declined. The expansion of jail beds in numerous counties in the U.S. sparked capitalist interest in utilization. Pretrial detentions have been on the rise. Residents from rural counties across the U.S. shared the burden and accounted for the 436% increase in pretrial detentions from the period of 1970–2013. Pretrial inmates consisted of two-thirds of the prison population. With diminutive resources, access to community services, prevention programs or the availability of judges to hear cases more frequently were constrained.

Eason (2012) acknowledged the realities of crime, poverty concentration and racial disadvantage was prevalent not only in urban spaces, but in rural locations as well. Nevertheless, the criminal justice literature neglected to map these connections. Dubbed, the rural ghetto or hyperghetto, Eason connected the possibility of high incarceration rates in these rural spaces were analogous to urban ghettos due to concentrated poverty. There was an array of evidence that proved this symbiotic relationship. African Americans disproportionately made up the inmate population and 72% of African Americans chose to reside in southern regions. In fact, the migration of blacks to rural areas reversed the typical composition of rural populations in some southern areas. During the decline of urban housing developments, rural public housing expanded and attracted poorer migrants to rural locales. Subsequently, researchers found parallels between rural and urban residential segregation and economic deprivation (Lichter and Brown 2011). Similar to challenges in urban communities with concentrated poverty, by the 1980s, crack became an epidemic in rural locales, violence escalated and resulted in the manifestation of prisoner reentry into rural areas. The highest incarceration rates were in southern states and criminal justice policies were more punitive and less rehabilitative in southern states.

To date, 60% of U.S. prisons are located in rural areas, mainly in predominantly Black and Hispanic areas. Initially, local residents objected planning initiatives for land use subjected to prison placement and proclaimed it had a negative impact on the rural economy. However, as ghetto characteristics emerged in rural locales, the preferences of rural elites re-framed collective action and supported prison placement. Whites benefited from employment in the prison industry and overrepresented the staff in rural prisons. However, Blacks and Hispanics in rural ghettos consisted of the same inhabitants as the prisons, which resulted in greater stigmatization, tension and marginalization in local rural communities. Eason (2012) eluded that considerations for prison placement was perhaps contingent on the racial and ethnic composition of the rural community.

Health Disparities in Prisoners

Prior research confirmed the adverse risks of inadequate health care and poorer health outcomes for people in the criminal justice system (Binswanger et al. 2009; Wilper et al. 2009). The differences in the healthcare systems of correctional facilities and the general population contributed to these outcomes and impacted the process and quality of health care delivery for inmates (Binswanger et al. 2012). The extent of chronic and infectious disease across racial and ethnic groups are not well known due to gaps in the research, mainly, from the exclusion of health conditions of inmates compared to the general population in national surveys (Wilper 2009). This creates a gross underestimation of disease prevalence in the U.S. However, given existing data, African Americans and minorities who were incarcerated have higher disease prevalence compared to non-incarcerated whites (Nkansah-Amankra 2013).

Studies showed that people with mental illnesses were not on their psychiatric medication at the time of arrest. Also, many inmates with a physical condition lacked continuity of care while in prison custody. The prison system is also renowned for its malicious treatment of inmates and reprehensible environment (Covin 2012).

Coordinated efforts between the correctional system and community health services for inmates transitioning back into the community could alleviate the risk of mortality linked to prison release (Rosen et al. 2008). Studies showed that men released from prison in North Carolina had a greater risk of death as a result of their vulnerability to injuries and medical conditions common in correctional facilities. In addition, this latter effort could also improve medication compliance. Given these aforementioned challenges, scholars offered alternative measures to decrease health disparities among inmates (Binswanger et al. 2017). Researchers recommended screening for infectious and chronic diseases that were prevalent among incarcerated populations upon prison entry, during custody, at the point of release and during the probationary period. Studies showed that these additive initiatives would control healthcare costs and improve public safety. However, federal policies restricted public funding for health care services for prisoners and financing was subjected to funds allocated from taxpayers.

Capitalism in the Criminal Justice System

According to French Sociologists Durkeim (1858–1917), poverty and deviance was considered a product of the social environment rather than a biological flaw. In a capitalist social order, poverty is inevitable and those who live in poverty were more likely to desire necessities and economic advantages, albeit from criminal activity (McCaghy et al. 2016). The class struggle embedded in capitalism created a subordinate class who sought refuge in illegal activities. Illegal methods were employed when the perception of opportunity was obstructed. Youth crime, particularly among boys in the lower economic strata, were at a disadvantage in conceptualizing middle class standards as attainable (Merton 1957). They found challenges in rhetoric that emphasized responsibility, ambition, and minimal aggression and found refuge in gang delinquency. Diminished accountability and compassion for others was abdicated in the pursuit to acquire the pleasures capitalist societies present. The interest of capitalists continues to factor into the literature when non-conformity to a social order resulted in any distress to wealthier classes, then, the act was considered punishable and prohibited. This is not to infer that the justice system is controlled by those who hold economic power, however, the system is subjected to the influence of certain groups.

Excessive incarceration rates among racial and ethnic groups is documented extensively in the criminal justice literature (Lofstrom and Raphael 2016). Uneducated African American men have a 70% greater chance of incarceration prior to their mid-thirties (Kearney et al. 2014). However, race and poverty are often juxtaposed and scientific evidence showed economic disadvantage posed an even greater risk of incarceration (Covin 2012). The U.S. prison system is overcrowded with individuals who are poor, lack power and non-property owners (Covin 2012). Individuals in the higher economic strata have committed more crimes, however, the poor, historically, received stricter adjudication. The inadequate ability to attain economic mobility was linked to criminalization in urban, inner city communities where the majority of residents were poor, homeless and suffered from mental illness and substance misuse. In this instance, the dissolution of social order in vulnerable communities can be applied to Rawls' theory of justice, which described the concept of reciprocity. Reciprocity involves a balanced exchange which leads to the subsequent presence of social cooperation and/or mutual benefit (Hartley 2014). His theory implied that if the most indigent populations had equitable access to good and services, this would afford them greater opportunities to alter their life trajectories from criminogenic choices (Covin 2012). Marginalized groups could make sufficient contributions that are aligned with society's values. In addition, dismantling policies that harshly penalized or profiled certain communities could alleviate incarceration rates among economically disadvantaged populations.

Neoliberalization in the U.S. is an ideology of laissez faire, diminutive state regulations, tax relief for the wealthy and follows up with the implementation of policies to support such principles (Nkansah-Amankra et al. 2013). The neoliberal capitalist social order, which is also noted as an accelerated form of profit maximization, shapes the outcomes of anti-poverty programs, the availability of public health initiatives and further aggravates incarceration rates, health disparities and economic inequalities (Nkansah-Amankra et al. 2013). The neoliberal agenda purports poverty through the devolution of investments in public welfare. Neoliberals regard this as a wasteful expenditure and criticized individuals who utilized these benefits. The valorization of capital is sovereign and market based policies were implemented to protect the interests of Corporations across all industries. This widened income inequality and exacerbated social unrest, including criminal activity, in the poorest regions in the U.S. Prior research confirmed this association between high crime rates, poverty and income inequality (Western et al. 2004). Rising unemployment rates for unskilled workers caused social unrest by unskilled workers. Consequently, racialized and income based arrests increased significantly.

Neoliberal policies and massive investments in the prison system occurred concurrently in the past three decades. Significant investments were made in technology, prison buildings, and the police force. The criminal justice system implemented more punitive, long-term consequences for minor offenses, especially drug offenses and low income and minorities, especially African Americans were targeted the most. Concomitantly, scholarly evidence demonstrated steady decreases in incarceration rates prior to this same time period. This begs the question of what actually occurred to prompt the mass proliferation of the prison industry? In the late 1990's the retrenchment of welfare benefits occurred under the Clinton Administration. At the same time, funding for corrections exceeded expenditures on food stamps and Aid to Families with Dependent Children. More children lived in poverty as a result during a rising period of capital productivity. Prisoners had a greater chance of living in poverty after release. Upon release, ex-inmates entered a vicious, yet structural, cycle of poverty. Former inmates lost access to social services which could alleviate poverty such as employment options, quality healthcare and education financing options. These resources would otherwise be available to them, however, individuals in the higher socioeconomic strata benefit the most. Therefore, a system is created that reproduces and guarantees an economically disadvantaged class. This select group of individuals had limited options to overcome poverty, which is not only tied to gradients in health outcomes (SES and poor health association), but also to gradients in criminal activity, such that the absolute poor suffers the greatest from arrests, sentencing and incarceration.

The term, prison industrial complex, describes the government and motivated interests of corporate investment in the prison industry (Alexander 2012). A number of Corporations operate for profit correctional and detention facilities including Corrections Corporations of America (Thompson 2012). Additional investors include AT&T, Sprint, American Express, and Allstate, just to name a few. The Capitalists intent is to minimize the cost of labor for productivity. This was easily accessible in the prison system. Government agencies, such as Immigration and Customs Enforcement (ICE) pay private prison Corporations $95 daily for detainees while the cost for supervision is only $14. In addition, Corporations favored convict leases over labor outside of prisons (Lichtenstein 1997). Once an inmate entered the correctional system, they were assigned employment and the exploitation of cheap labor was readily available to capitalists. Textile companies and furniture factories employed prisoners. In the free world, textile workers earned $10.95 per hour and furniture factory workers earned $13.04 per hour while prisoners earned between .12 and $1.15 per hour to produce these same services. State wages for prisoner services were lower and range from $.13 to .32.

Consequently, private prisons had more safety violations, higher exposure to toxic metals, larger inmate to officer ratios and weekly work for prisoners were more extensive compared to government owned prisons. Corporations, therefore, were incentivized by mass incarceration and long term sentencing, even for minor offenses. The American Legislative Exchange Council (ALEC) served as the political lobbyists to protect Corporate profit seeking interests in the prison industry. Corporations, including Walmart, Hewlett Packard, McDonalds and private prisons joined the ALEC and spent millions advocating for harsh sentencing and jailing on capitol hill. By 2008, 2.3 million adults were in the custody of correctional facilities at the local, state and federal levels and 5.1 million were on probation or parole (Congressional Research Service 2010). This equated to a 400% boost in the prison population in the past few decades for arrests associated with drug laws, re-arrests, re-convictions or re-incarceration of ex-offenders.

Conclusion: Political Economy, Capitalism, Health and Rural Crime

Social disorder in rural locales have been both inadequate and punitive. With insufficient resources for substance abuse programs, drug misuse will continue to escalate. In rural areas, the scant supply of legal staff contributes to long term detainment in prisons.

The unique needs of this population requires public policy responses at the federal and state levels that are inclusive such that the needs of both urban and rural constituents are met. Public policies should abdicate neoliberal ideologies if the elimination of social unrest and health disparities in rural areas is the intention.

Rural communities face the daunting challenge of achieving economic mobility and prosperity. In the wake of depleting resources coupled with a lack of political will to enhance social services, rural communities are at greater risks of mortality, morbidity and overall, greater health disparities. With a neoliberal political agenda, this further exacerbates social discontent in rural areas and provokes a social disorder, not historically common in rural areas, leading to unprecedented arrests especially in rural communities.

The rural mystique is a far cry from its symbolic undertones. This chapter shows that the dissolution of social order in rural communities have long been ignored. Scholarship on incarceration patterns was largely segregated to the urban landscape while causation for rural imprisonments were discounted. Rural communities have been subjected to a neoliberal-capitalist society and the aftereffect is community breakdown and distress. The absence of goods and services not only impedes access to community services and programs, but it restricts access to economic mobility, which, in turn creates the propensity for criminogenic choices. With incarceration rates rising among rural residents, this further widens the health disparity gap between rural and urban populations. To construct a rural mystique requires a commitment to economic stability, infrastructure development, employment opportunities and investment in social programs.

References

Alexander, M. (2012). *The new jim crow: Mass incarcerations in the age of colorblindness.* New York: The New Press.

Binswanger, I. A., Krueger, P. M., & Steiner, J. F. (2009). Prevalence of chronic medical conditions among jail and prison inmates in the USA compared with the general population. *Journal of Epidemiology and Community Health, 63*(11), 912–919.

Binswanger, I. A., Redmond, N., Steiner, J. F., & Hicks, L. S. (2012). Health disparities and the criminal justice system: An agenda for further research and action. *Journal of Urban Health: Bulletin of the New York Academy of Medicine, 89*(1), 98–107. https://doi.org/10.1007/s11524-011-9614-1.

Binswanger, I. A., Blatchford, P. J., Forsyth, S. J., Stern, M. F., & Kinner, S. A. (2016). Epidemiology of infectious disease–related death after release from prison, Washington State, United States, and Queensland, Australia: A Cohort Study. *Public Health Reports, 131*(4), 574–582.

Brown, D., & Schafft, K. (2011). *Rural people and communities in the 21st century.* Malden: Polity Press.

Can, S. (2014). *Collective efficacy.* https://doi.org/10.1002/9781118517383.wbeccj285. Retrieved from: file://www.home/chronos/u-19866ab2fee2dfd5adc206fdc21bf2c2ae18bd2a/Downloads/Collective%20Efficacy,d285.pdf

Congressional Research Service. (2010). *Economic impacts of prison growth.* Retrieved from: https://fas.org/sgp/crs/misc/R41177.pdf

Covin, L. (2012). Homelessness, poverty, and incarceration: The criminalization of despair. *Journal of Forensic Psychology Practice, 12*(5), 439–456.

Deller, S. C., & Deller, M. A. (2010). Rural crime and social capital. *Growth and Change, 41*(2), 221–275.

Donnermeyer, J. (2007). Rural crime: Roots and restoration. *International Journal of Rural Crime, 1*, 2–20.

Eason, J. M. (2012). Extending the Hyperghetto: Toward a theory of punishment, race, and rural disadvantage. *Journal of Poverty, 16*(3), 274.

Gottfredson, M., & Hirschi, T. (1990). *A general theory of crime*. Stanford: Stanford UP.

Harbeck, K. M. (2015). *Social disorganization theory*. Research starters: Sociology (Online Edition).

Hartley, C. (2014). Two conceptions of justice as reciprocity. *Social Theory and Practice, 40*(3), 409.

Jones, J. (2012). Looking beyond the 'rural idyll': Some recent trends in rural crime. *Criminal Justice Matters, 89*(1), 8–9.

Kang-Brown, J, & Subramanian, R. (2017). *Out of sight: The growth of jails in rural America*. New York: Vera Institute of Justice. Retrieved from: http://www.safetyandjusticechallenge.org/wp-content/uploads/2017/06/Out_of_sight_report.pdf

Kaylen, M. T., & Pridemore, W. A. (2013). Social disorganization and crime in rural communities: A first direct test of the systemic model. The. *British Journal of Criminology, 53*, 905–923.

Kearney, M. Harris, B. Jacome, E., & Parker, L. (2014). *The Hamilton project: Ten economic facts about crime and incarceration in the United States*. Retrieved from: https://www.brookings.edu/wp-content/uploads/2016/06/v8_THP_10CrimeFacts.pdf

Lee, M., & Ousey, G. (2001). Size matters: Examining the link between small manufacturing, socioeconomic deprivation, and crime rates in nonmetropolitan communities. *Sociological Quarterly, 42*(4), 581.

Lichtenstein, A. (1997). *Twice the work of free labor: The political economy of convict labor in the New South*. New York: Verso.

Lichter, D., & Brown, D. (2011). Rural America in an urban society: Changing spatial and social boundaries. *Annual Review of Sociology, 37*, 565–592.

Lofstrom, M., & Raphael, S. (2016). Crime, the criminal justice system, and socioeconomic inequality. *Journal of Economic Perspectives, 30*(2), 103–126.

McCaghy, C., Capron, T., Jamieson, J., Harley, S., & Carey, H. (2016). *Deviant behavior: Crime, conflict, and interest groups* (8th ed.). New York: Routledge Taylor & Francis Group.

McGranahan, D. (1986). *Crime and the countryside. Rural development perspectives*. Retrieved from: https://naldc.nal.usda.gov/download/AGE86927751/PDF

Merton, R. K. (1957). *Social theory and social structure*, revised and enlarged edition. New York: Free Press of Glencoe.

Miller, S. (1976). The political economy of social problems: From the sixties to the seventies. *Social Problems, 24*(1), 131–141.

Moore, M., & Sween, M. (2015). Rural youth crime: A reexamination of social disorganization theory's applicability to rural areas. *Journal of Juvenile Justice, 4*(1), 47–63.

Nkansah-Amankra, S., Kwami Agbanu, S., & Miller, R. (2013). Disparities in health, poverty, incarceration, and social justice among racial groups in the United States: A critical review of evidence of close links with neoliberalism. *International Journal of Health Services, 43*(2), 217–240.

Reichert, C., Cromartie, J., & Arthun, R. (2014). Reasons for returning and not returning to rural U.S. communities. *The Professional Geographer, 66*(1), 58–72.

Rosen, D. L., Schoenbach, V. J., & Wohl, D. A. (2008). All-cause and cause-specific mortality among men released from state prison, 1980–2005. *American Journal of Public Health, 98*(12), 2278–2284.

Shaw, C. R., & McKay, H. D. (1942). *Juvenile delinquency and urban areas*. Chicago: University of Chicago Press.

Shihadeh, E. S., & Barranco, R. E. (2010). Latino employment and non-Latino homicide in rural areas: The implications of U.S. immigration policy. *Deviant Behavior, 31*(5), 411–439.

Soukhanov, A. (Ed.). (2004). *Ecology. Encarta Webster's dictionary of the English language* (2nd ed.). New York: Bloomsbury.

The National Center for Victims on Crime. (2017). *Urban and rural victimization.* Retrieved from: https://victimconnect.org/wp-content/uploads/2015/09/2017NCVRW_UrbanRural_Final.pdf

Thomas, W. I., & Znaniecki, F. W. ([1918–1920] 1996). *The polish peasant in Europe and America: Monograph of an Immigrant Group.* Urbana: University of Illinois Press. ISBN 0252064844

Thompson, H. (2012). The prison industrial complex: A growth industry in a shrinking economy. *New Labor Forum, 21*(3), 39–47.

Weisheit, R., Falcone, D., & Wells, L. (2006). *Crime and policing in rural and small-town America.* Long Grove: Waveland Press.

Wells, L. E., & Weisheit, R. A. (2004). Patterns of rural and urban crime: A county-level comparison. *Criminal Justice Review, 29*(1), 1–22.

Western, B., Rosenfeld, J, & Kleykamp, M. (2004). *Economic inequality and the rise in U.S. imprisonment.* Retrieved from: https://www.russellsage.org/sites/all/files/u4/Western,%20 Kleykamp,%20%26%20Rosenfeld_Economic%20Inequality%20and%20the%20Rise%20 in%20US%20Imprisonment.pdf

Wilper, A. P., Woolhandler, S., Boyd, J. W., et al. (2009). The health and health care of US prisoners: Results of a nationwide survey. *American Journal of Public Health, 99*, 666–672.

Chapter 4
Political Economy in the Era of Trump Politics

Capitalism is embedded in the U.S. economic system. There are categories of capitalism that reflect specific types of political regimes. For example, political regimes (or political administrations) can be considered economic or extra- economic in the context of capitalism (Jessop 2002). Governmentality is then based on an economic articulation expressed through macroeconomic policies that support such ideologies. The distinction between economic and an extra-economic order reproduces either regulated or deregulated markets, determines the degree of competitiveness in global markets, and any shifts in capital accumulation, that is, accelerated capital production or capital reinvestment in social welfare.

Keynesian Welfare National State (KWNS) and Schumpeterian Workfare State (SWS) are two distinct models of economic development theories that exist in a capitalist society (Jessop 2002). Governments that endorse Keynesian economics believe free markets require regulation given its fluctuations during periods of economic instability, i.e. recessions. Other features of KWNS include the mass production of semi-skilled labour, income increases, profits, investments and wages. With government intervention, Keynesian economics balances conflicts between supply and demand for public goods, capitalism and labour, full employment and endorses welfare provisions with social policies aimed to promote economic growth and earnings for all citizens. The manifestations of Keynesian economics in politics is represented in a social contract committed to redistributive policies. Schumpeterian economics assumes extra economic conditions in which complete reliance on free markets are valued. SWS defends its accelerated pursuit for capital accumulation within and outside U.S. borders as fundamental to economic growth. SWS' competitive nature embraces new innovations and technology with consideration of regenerating or replacing old industries. Neoliberal globalized markets are fiscally advantageous to capitalists. Profit maximization is a key feature under the SWS along with the belief that such profits will eventually trickle down and benefit poorer populations. Political administrations with a Schumpeterian framework authenticate policies towards

© The Author(s) 2018
M. M. Taylor, *Application of the Political Economy to Rural Health Disparities*,
SpringerBriefs in Public Health, https://doi.org/10.1007/978-3-319-73537-5_4

economic intervention versus government intervention, underscores public and private partnerships and regards social policies as subservient to the needs of extra economic conditions.

Formal knowledge of the type of economic order of political administrations is essential to understand the type of policies that can be expected when a candidate is sworn into the Presidency. In this current political era, we can evaluate if President Trump's political agenda, emulates Keynesian or Schumpeterian theory. Using such theories, we are able to assess if Trump's political agenda demonstrates a commitment towards improving the welfare of *Rural* or *Corporate* America. An assessment of the existing polity helps to predetermine what the quality of life could be for rural populations, during and after the Trump Era. Rural America demonstrated overwhelming support for President Trump in the 2016 elections (Leonard 2017; Evich 2016). Trump made many promises during his campaign – promises that the best interest of rural America would be served upon his election as President. He campaigned to improve conditions in rural communities and used common rhetoric on issues that concerned rural populations including population loss, trade deals and the decline of the American farmer in the labor market. The Conservative, pro-religious base in rural America found Trump's messaging appealing and in insurmountable numbers, and without concrete rural policies attached, rural America voted for the newly elected president.

The electoral outcome of the Trump nomination reflected constituents who had lower incomes and less education compared to voters for Hillary Clinton (Manuel 2017). Given this, an assessment of Trump's rural policy plans are significant to determine if his agenda, will indeed, benefit the welfare of this group. Below, are select policies to of consideration.

Immigration Reform

Background

Approximately 244 million persons do not reside in their country of origin (Parmet et al. 2017). The U.S. houses the largest number of immigrants in the world and by 2014, 13.2% of the population were immigrants, with only 3.5% undocumented. In the U.S., young undocumented immigrants were able to obtain temporary legal status through the Deferred Action for Childhood Arrivals (DACA) legislation passed in 2012 under the Obama Administration (Institute on Taxation and Economic Policy 2017). These young, undocumented immigrants migrated to the U.S. with their parents and enrollment in DACA deferred their deportation and gave them legal status to work in the U.S. These young immigrants pay approximately 2 billion dollars annually in state and local taxes. Overall, the U.S. economy benefited by greater than $11.74 billion dollars from the 11 million working, undocumented, young immigrants. DACA enrollees are employed in various industries and currently pays a higher portion of their income towards taxes compared to the top 1%

earners, at 8.9% and 5.4% respectively. Their tax dollars finance public infrastructure and the schools systems in the communities they reside in. Immigrants, however, are less likely to have insurance due to their employment in jobs that do not offer employer sponsored health insurance or because their status excludes them from acquiring public benefits. Historically, and in error, immigrants were often blamed for disease outbreaks that occurred in the U.S.

Trump Agenda

The Trump Administration made the decision to rescind the DACA program in September of 2017 claiming that immigration prevented native-born residents from obtaining employment and also accounted for higher unemployment rates among African Americans and Latinos (U.S. Department of Justice 2017; Jan 2017). In addition, the Administration claimed that immigration put our nation at risk for crime and violence and the decision to phase out DACA in an attempt to restore a constitutional order in America on the immigration process. However, there is insufficient evidence that shows that immigration substantially impedes employment for native-born residents (Stone 2017; Jan 2017). The effect of immigration, albeit minimal, is experienced by native born high school dropouts or by low skilled immigrant workers. Research supports evidence that immigration boosts the economy with highly skilled immigrants demonstrating a positive effect on the earnings of native born Americans. The challenge with the Trump Administration's claims on DACA participants limiting employment for minorities is further arguable since the skills, experience and education levels of unemployed minorities in the DACA age group may not be comparable. DACA participants are more likely to be college educated and typically pursue quality employment. In addition, immigration reform rhetoric under the current Administration has been commonly associated with criminality, during a era where deportation of criminals increased to 80%. Consequently, the focus should rest on the salient potential for educated immigrants to contribute to society.

Rescinding the DACA program would result in a loss of state and local taxes by approximately $800 million dollars and cause a reduction in annual contributions to 1.2 billion (Institute on Taxation and Economic Policy 2017). States would experience substantial losses in economic contributions from DACA participants, including California whose 379,000 participants contribute $534 million, Florida's 72,000 young immigrants contribute over $100 million, New York's 76,000 participants contribute over $140 million, and in Texas, their 177,000 participants contribute over $313 million to the states' economy. Many economists find Trump's decision to phase out the program economically, unsubstantiated, especially since programs to establish paths to citizenship would add approximately $505 million to state and local taxes and increase annual revenues, overall, to nearly $2.53 billion. Many of America's Companies, including Amazon, Google, AT&T, Wells Fargo, Microsoft and Apple, have advocated to protect DACA participants from being deported (Hincks 2017).

Notwithstanding the abundance of economic evidence from many economists on DACA's benefits, phasing out the DACA program would also burden the economy. The process to execute Trump's decision will result in mass deportations, costing the U.S. $12,500 to retain each undocumented DACA participant (Stone 2017).

Impact on Rural America

Approximately 1.8 million youths are undocumented and a quarter of this population (252,000) have taken residences in rural towns (Kissam 2012). Most are farmworkers and have Spanish descent. Texas has the highest concentration of DACA eligible immigrants with farming skills, followed by North Carolina, Florida, Arizona and Georgia.

While immigration is largely prevalent across nations, expressions of xenophobia persists, rather cogently, including in rural populations. Rural populations in the U.S. mostly have a negative perception on immigration (Altman 2016; HJKFF 2017a). They depict immigrants as a burden on this country. However, rural economies have prospered from the influx of immigrants to this region and reversed trends in population depreciation (Center for Rural Affairs 2017). Farming opportunities and production increased and credit lines for Latino owned businesses in rural towns bolstered the rural economy. Without opportunities to enroll in the DACA program, many of these young immigrants were less likely to pursue a college education or higher paying jobs (Kissam 2012).

The economic contributions of DACA participants have also been instrumental in restoring economic growth in rural areas (Joint Economic Committee 2017). The 91% of DACA participants that live in rural communities are employed. The majority of rural beneficiaries of DACA are employed in careers that align with their long term goals and 61% of them have jobs where they can acquire health insurance benefits after enrollment in DACA. Approximately 5% became entrepreneurs after they enrolled in the program. Seventy percent of rural beneficiaries reported that they were able to support their families after being accepted in the program and 22% became first time home owners in their rural communities.

In addition to legislative changes to DACA, Trump's revised executive order to ban travel and block issuances on new visas to migrants from Iran, Sudan, Somalia, Libya, Syria and Yemen, which was signed in January of 2017, impacted the medical industry (McGraw et al. 2017). Over 25% of physicians that practiced medicine in the U.S. were impacted by Trump's travel ban because they were foreign born (Minier 2017). Approximately 7000 foreign born physicians practice in rural and underserved areas – areas where native born physicians are not amenable to accept. Annually, 14 million doctors visits were administered by foreign born physicians to patients in a designated Health Professional Shortage Areas. Many national organizations such as the American College of Physicians and the Association of American Medical Colleges opposed the ban due to the barriers it posed to access healthcare to vulnerable communities and its restrictions on issuing visas to international students to pursue a medical education in the U.S (AAMC 2017; American College of Physicians 2017). These organizations urged President Trump to exercise discretion and waive the travel ban and visas for international medical graduates, physicians and researchers. By June of 2017, amendments were made such that persons with existing academic, familial and job connections were excluded from the travel ban (McGraw et al. 2017).

In September of 2017, the President continued to engage in discussions with Congress to phase out DACA in the next 6 months (Newman 2017). This would leave a dearth in the healthcare workforce since one fifth of DACA's beneficiaries work in this industry. The rural economy would suffer tremendously and the trend toward population loss would persist. The impact of the broken family unit cannot be measured economically and the diversity in rural communities including the skills and talent in the workforce would be affected the most and in the absence of significant interest group pressure on the President's travel ban, there would have been an even greater shortage of physicians in rural areas.

Prison Industrial Complex: Revisited

As discussed in Chap. 3, the prison industrial complex resulted in a rise of incarcerations centered on drug related crimes and a progression in incarcerations among rural residents. Federal (and state) laws such as the Sentencing Reform Act of 1984 and the Anti Drug Abuse Act of 1986, precipitated policing.

The Sentencing Reform Act (SRA) was adopted to ensure uniformity in jail sentences for similar crimes in Federal cases (Howell 2004). The Sentencing Guidelines Commission was established for the determination of the extent of jail time for adult felonies, which included violent, sex and drug offenders. Prior to the passage of the SRA, Courts had full discretion on sentencing structure for offenses. The SRA rejected rehabilitation in sentencing considerations and revoked the possibility for parole. Judges also had accountability and had to document their rationale for the sentences they rendered. To date, the SRA has not been grandfathered for sentences that occurred prior to 1984. Since the policy was implemented in 1984, the prison population doubled in Washington (Washington State Sentencing Guidelines Commission 2017).

Growing political pressure emerged on the sentencing disparities in the SRA (Howell 2004). In response to the opposition and claims of injustices under the SRA, President Bush signed into law, the Feeney Amendment to the Prosecutorial Remedies and Tools Against the Exploitation of Children Today Act of 2003. Research statistics on trial judges demonstrated that they were still not executing uniformity on mandatory sentencing laws. Hence, the PROTECT ACT was passed to further increase equity in sentencing structure and created fewer opportunities for judges to exercise discretion. This policy also required additional documentation from judges on sentencing decisions.

The Anti-Drug Abuse Act required time served in jail for illegal possession of drugs or drug trafficking (American Civil Liberties Union 2006). Harsher mandatory 5 year sentences was imposed for possession of 5 g of crack cocaine. However, 500 g of powdered cocaine carried the same prison sentence. This law posed greater sentencing disparities because crack cocaine was more afford-able to poor Americans, especially African Americans. Powdered cocaine was more likely utilized by wealthy white Americans. Research showed that African Americans were unjustly punished for crack cocaine offenses compared to White defendants. When drug crimes continued to rise, Congress enacted the Omnibus Anti-Drug Abuse Act of 1988. This law imposed a 5 year minimum and 20 year maximum on drug possession that included in excess of 5 g or more of crack cocaine.

More recently, anti-immigrant bias, emerging immigration labor policies and stereotypical perceptions of immigrants as criminals incited massive forms of policing which led to increased detentions and deportations, particularly among Latino immigrants, creating the *Immigration Industrial Complex* (Diaz 2011). Federal policies were implemented after immigrant labor was used in various indus-tries. For example, the Chinese population aided in the construction of railroads, Filipinos, Japanese and Mexicans tiled fields and when their labor was completed, legislation was passed to restrict their presence in the U.S. Federal policies such as E-verify, which restricts companies from employing unauthorized immigrants and No Match Letters, where Employers are informed by the IRS of employees without social security numbers, qualified immigrants as felons or subject to depor-tation (National Immigration Law Center 2009; U.S. Citizenship and Immigration Services 2017).

Historically, immigrants depicted as criminals were arrested and deported back to their country of origin. However, contemporary policing measures fueling the Immigration Industrial Complex detained immigrants in privately owned prisons who profited substantially from immigrant arrests (Diaz 2011). Undocumented Latinos were disproportionately subjected to workplace arrests and imprisonment, which was instigated by Federal policies. Immigrant detainment increased from 6785 in 1995 to 22,000 in 2006.

To date, the Trump Administration sought to expand its capacity to house prison-ers for deportations (Richardson 2017). His immigration reform goals will require added jail occupancies. The White House budget allocated billions towards new jails for immigrant detainees. Over 97,000 people suspicious of illegal immigration status have been arrested from the period of January 2017 to September of 2017. Stock prices for private prison owners (Corrections Corporation of America) rose substantially after Trump was elected into office (Surowiecki 2016). In addition, appeals from the Obama Justice Department for the Trump Administration to elimi-nate the use of private prison facilities have been abdicated.

Impact on Rural America

Given the economic evidence described in this section, President Trump's decision to end the DACA program will *hurt* rural America and would lead to higher imprisonment rates for rural America. Massive, non-criminal immigrants would essentially be detained in prisons until they are deported to their country of origin. The President's goals are contrary to both public and political will. Bipartisan bills were introduced to Congress for the past 2 years on sentencing reform by Senators Grassley (Republican, Iowa) and Durbin (Democrat, Illinois) in an effort to reduce the prison population (Committee on the Judiciary 2017). The Sentencing Reform and Corrections Act of 2017 proposes to decrease prison sentences for nonviolent drug offenses and subject only violent drug crimes to mandatory minimum sentences. In addition, Judges could retroactively reduce jail time for persons with long term sentences as a result of disparities between crack and cocaine trafficking.

The president's political agenda on immigration reform does not advance or benefit the lives of rural Americans, but rather criminalize a vulnerable population. Rural populations will continue to endure mass incarcerations for minor offenses under existing federal laws, and if DACA is phased out, a substantial amount of detainments of rural immigrants is anticipated, causing rural populations to further, overpopulate the prison system.

Personal Protection and Affordable Care Act

Background

The Affordable Care Act was implemented to expand health insurance coverage to citizens and legal residents in an effort to reduce the uninsured population in America (HJKFF 2017b). The uninsured rate dropped from nearly 44 million in 2013 to 28 million by the end of 2016. Many still lacked health insurance due to the high costs of coverage, were ineligible through their employers, change in family status or resided in states that did not participate in Medicaid expansion. Disparities in the uninsured rate remain in African American and Hispanics.

Geographically, rural residents were disproportionately affected by state laws to abdicate Medicaid expansion (HJKFF 2017c). Nearly two-thirds of the rural population resided in these states. Healthcare coverage was particularly challenging in rural populations compared to metropolitan residents because they were generally poorer, which made paying for insurance inaccessible. Public insurance was more prevalent among rural residents and given the type of low paying jobs available in rural areas, they were less likely to acquire insurance through an employer compared to their urban counterparts. Three out of four rural residents met the income eligibility requirements to receive tax credits under the ACA, however, without state participation in Medicaid expansion, many rural groups had fewer options for coverage. Medicaid offers little options as many rural residents exceeded the eligibility levels.

The ACA was instrumental in bringing financial assistance to rural hospitals. The Balanced Budget Act of 1997, section 402 implemented provisions for a Critical Access Hospital (CAH) designation for rural healthcare facilities (American Hospital Association 2016). This designation was intended to prevent financial risk of hospital closures in rural areas. Rural hospitals with 25 or fewer inpatient beds, located at least 35 miles from another hospital and provided 24 h emergency care received this designation. CAHs were eligible for Medicare reimbursements. These provisions were extended to hospitals that had a non-profit and for-profit status.

However, economic instability resulted in closures for 66 rural hospitals (NCSL 2017). By March of 2016, some 673 hospitals still posed a risk of closure and 68% of these hospital were CAHs. These hospitals have been burdened by a lack of support from states to participate in Medicaid expansion.

In addition, the Rural Community Hospital Demonstration program (RCHD) provides cost-based reimbursements to large hospitals in rural areas that do not have the designation of a Critical Access Hospital (Centers for Medicare and Medicaid Services 2017a, b). This program was originally initiated under the Medicare Modernization Act of 2003. The ACA enacted provisions to extend the program until October 1st, 2017 and more recently, Section 15003 of the twenty-first Century Cure Act proposed to extend the RCHD program for an additional 10 years.

The purpose and benefit of the ACA for improving access to healthcare in rural populations is clear-cut. If any parts of the ACA provisions are repealed, the economic viability of rural hospitals could result in additional closures and approximately 700,000 rural residents could lose access to emergency room care.

Trump's Agenda

Trump's proposed bill, the American Health Care Act, was designed to replace parts of the ACA which directly affect the Federal budget (Davis 2017; Willison and Singer 2017). Mandatory provisions for employers, various taxes and the individual mandate clause were retracted in Trump's proposal. If Trump's policy is passed, by 2026, approximately 23 million people will be uninsured due to the following: (1) people with pre-existing conditions are not afforded protections; (2) retrenchment of subsidies to support low income persons; (3) retrenchment of Medicaid expansion; and (4) insurance premiums will increase to 60% and presumed unaffordable to many. If the bill is passed, states have the option to waive the minimal requirement for essential health benefits. Over a 10 year period, the American Health Care Act would cut the deficit by $119 billion. However, the plan would consist of over $830 billion in cuts to Medicaid. The bill passed in the House of Representatives and the Senate is now redrafting a new version of the bill. Although Republicans hold the majority vote in the Senate, they could not reach a consensus on Trump's version of health care reform.

Impact on Rural America

The ACA expanded coverage to people in rural areas, which, in turn, generated revenue for rural hospitals (Luthra 2017). Revenues in rural hospitals increased 33% since 2013 in Medicaid expansion states compared to merely 1.1% in non expansion states (Broaddus 2017). Rural hospitals in states that expanded Medicaid had a 43% decrease in their utilization of uncompensated care costs compared to the 16% in non-expansion states. Repealing Medicaid expansion would cause rural hospitals to incur bad debts (for patients unable to pay) and create a further financial hardship on these institutions if comparable policy provisions are not implemented. Rural hospitals have a long-term history of financial crisis leading to many facility closures and some still at risk. Medicaid expansion provided financial stability to facilities at risk for closure.

Pennsylvania has a large rural population, third in the country, and this was a key voting state in the Trump election (Luthra 2017). In fact, 64% of the people in Fayette County, which is one of Pennsylvania's poorest counties, voted for President Trump, When the ACA was implemented, 625,000 people acquired insurance in Pennsylvania and nearly half of these enrollees (300,000) were from the states' rural population. Many were not aware that their expanded coverage for prescriptions and added benefits were the result of ACA provisions. Rural hospitals in Pennsylvania profited the most, from the provisions in the ACA, due to their higher capacity of poor and sicker patients in the rural parts of the state. Fayette County, in particularly, ranks among the lowest in health outcomes relative to other counties in the state. Nearly a third of the population are obese, they experience higher rates of drug overdoses and nearly one in ten have diabetes.

Overall, rural populations gained insurance coverage in states that participated in Medicaid expansion (HJKFF 2017d). The uninsured rate dropped significantly among rural americans. Between 2013 and 2015, two million rural Americans enrolled in the ACA in key Republican states. In Pennsylvania, the rural uninsured rate decreased from 13% (2013) to 8% (2015); Michigan 15% (2013) to 8% (2015), Ohio 14% (2013) to 8%(2015); and Iowa 11% (2013) to 6% (2015). Each of these states were formerly democratic, but voted Republican in the 2016 elections. Of the states that expanded medicaid, 17 had Republican governors compared to 13 Democratic governors (HJKFF 2017c). The uninsured rates for the former, would increase substantially if ACA provisions are repealed. Rural populations in states that did not participate in Medicaid expansion only experienced a 1% increase in Medicaid coverage between 2013 and 2015 (Foutz et al. 2017).

By far, a repeal of the ACA would *hurt* rural populations. Any replacement of the ACA that does not include equal or greater Medicaid provisions will *hurt* existing rural healthcare facilities at risk for closure. Republican districts will suffer the greatest with 5.9 million ACA enrollees compared to the 5.2 million that reside in Democratic states (HJKFF 2017e).

Medicaid and State Children's Health Insurance Program

Background

The Children's Health Insurance Program was implemented as a provision in the Balanced Budget Act of 1997 to allocate Medicaid funding to expand coverage for low income children (HJKFF 1997). With over 10 million children uninsured during that time, children who were 19 and younger whose families income met the eligibility requirements were covered under CHIP The program has been reauthorized a few times with moderate provisions. More importantly, the uninsured rate for children dropped from 14% in 1997 to 5% in 2016 (HJKFF 2017f). Each state expanded coverage to increase coverage eligibility for children under CHIP. CHIP is the second largest source of health insurance coverage for children in the U.S. In 2015, 53% of the children in the U.S. were covered by Employer Sponsored Health Insurance or private insurance and 39% were covered through Medicaid/CHIP. In 2017, nearly 9 million children are covered under CHIP. In the absence of funding for CHIP, states would bear the financial burden to offer insurance protections for children.

Trump Agenda

Trump's proposed budget plan includes a retrenchment of programs that directly benefit the poor. The proposed American Health Care Act will restructure Medicaid. This would entail placing limits on federal funding for expenditures associated with Medicaid, including CHIP. Funding for CHIP expired on September 30, 2017, however, in December, Congress extended funding for the CHIP program to states who were most at risk for depleting their funds before the end of December of 2017 (Quinn 2017). In October, Arizona, California, Minnesota, Washington and Oregon received federal funding to extend CHIP. Other states are preparing options to extend funding, however, 16 states will exhaust their funding sources by early 2018 in the absence of federal assistance (HJKFF 2017g). These short term solutions does not guarantee CHIP would be reauthorized in 2018. Trump's budget for Medicaid is projected to be cut by over $800 billion, which could impact continuity in funding for CHIP.

Impact on Rural America

Historically, rural children had significantly higher uninsured rates compared to urban children. Medicaid and The Children's Health Insurance Program helped to narrow this gap in geographical disparity (Mueller et al. 2012; O'Hare 2007).

Since CHIP's inception, rural children were 18% less likely than urban children to become uninsured. Research studies show that rural children rely more on CHIP or Medicaid coverage compared to urban children. This is primarily due to the disproportionate number of low income families that reside in rural areas who meet the program's eligibility requirements.

Prior to CHIP, 19% of rural children were uninsured compared to 16% urban children. These rates dropped significantly during the period of 2003–2007 where only 12% of rural children were uninsured compared to urban children at 14%. By 2009, CHIP/Medicaid covered 40% of rural children compared to 32% of urban children. This evidence demonstrates that Medicaid/CHIP has been a critical safety net for Rural America, especially rural children. Medicaid has been an instrumental source to supplement the gap in coverage in rural america, who have fewer access to employment and employer sponsored health insurance compared to their urban counterparts. In the absence of continued funding for CHIP or if significant cuts to Medicaid are realized, this would *hurt* rural America. For rural America, access to care is pivotal in the reduction of excessive emergency room visits, morbidity and premature mortality.

Tax Reform Policy

Background

The tax code in the United States has been, historically, problematic. Tax systems should consist of enough dividends sufficient for government expenditures (Gale and Krupkin 2016). Economists suggest alleviating the tax burden from middle and low income households to higher income households could correct the tax code. Tax policies have historically, benefitted households with larger incomes due to specific provisions to offset tax deductions and exemptions (Bernstein 2013). Consequently, middle and lower income earners are not afforded equal tax incentives as higher income households for similar deductions, i.e. home purchases. Reconstructing the corporate income tax and increasing revenues to counterbalance America's financial deficit was also recommended to improve the U.S. tax system (Gale and Krupkin 2016). The existing corporate income tax system has some ambiguity because the source of corporate income and the residence of the corporation is not clearly defined (Toder and Viard 2014). More importantly, foreign source income from multinational corporations is not clear-cut and taxes on their profits are often deferred by foreign subsidiaries (Jared 2013). Multinationals, therefore, have a greater incentive to reinvest their profits globally or operate in nations with lower taxes, which further abdicates revenue from the U.S. economy. Finally, economists suggested a reduction in tax expenditures would raise revenues. However, there is a lack of consensus on which programs should receive less funding or get repealed, especially when such programs primarily support lower income families.

Trump Agenda

Tax reform under the Trump Administration favors corporations, multinationals and higher income earners (Huang et al. 2017). Corporations will experience a tax cut of 21% in 2018 from its historical 35% tax rate. Taxes on multinational corporations will have even more tax breaks on their foreign profits. While Trump's tax reform does include revenue increases, these increases are not enough to cover the costs applied to cuts in corporate taxes. By 2025, higher income earners will experience the highest tax cuts compared to people who make less than 30,000 annually. The latter, including people who make less than $75,000 annually would experience a large tax increases by 2027. Households with incomes greater than $40,000 will realize a positive change in their after tax income. Households with incomes between $40,000 and $50,000 will see a .3% change in their after tax income by 2025 compared to households with incomes between $500,000 and $1 million, who will receive a 2.4% increase in income. Households with incomes below $30,000 are worse off in Trump's tax reform policy. These earners will either have no change in their after tax income or their after tax income will be reduced in the long run.

The tax cuts on wealthy earners will ultimately add to America's deficit by $1.5 trillion.

In addition, in order to balance the cuts in corporate tax, the individual mandate in the ACA was repealed. This mandate required all persons to acquire health insurance or pay a penalty. The permanent repeal of this ACA provision, not only places a risk of 13 million persons falling on the uninsured rolls, but it also serves to subsidize one-third of the corporate tax rate.

Impact on Rural America

In the long run, President Trump's tax reform policy will *hurt* rural America. In order to subsidize the permanent tax cuts for millionaires and billionaires, a reduction in spending on social programs is mandatory. These programs benefit rural households. Tax cuts on wealthy Americans are offset by revenue generated from taxpayers, primarily from the lower income stratum. Poorer households are disproportionately located in rural areas and these households will receive less money in their after tax income, over the long run.

Trump Governance: Schumpeterian or Keynesian?

The political economy in the Trump era reflects policies that counter the well being of rural populations. The President's decision to phase out DACA, impacts population stability in rural areas as well as the rural economy. Many economists find

Trump's decision puzzling, given the insurmountable evidence that shows DACA enrollees contribute significantly to America's economy. To some degree, the Trump Administration's intention is illustrative of an extra-economic motivation to accelerate revenues in other areas, particularly for the (private) prison industry. The prison industry would realize substantial profits if DACA participants are policed and detained in private prisons.

Public expenditures to establish insurance coverage for America's most vulnerable populations was defrayed by permanent provisions for tax cuts to the wealthy and corporations. In addition, the Administration's failure to reauthorize CHIP by the programs' deadline raises ongoing concerns for access to healthcare for children. Rural adults and children would suffer the most, given their greater reliance on public insurance compared to their urban counterparts.

The advancement of capital proved to be cardinal to the existing political institution and further hinders economic mobility for non-capitalists. The broader myriad of policies, economic in nature, are described in this chapter and eventually shapes the lack of opportunities for investments in health policies that benefit rural populations. The economic policies promoted in the Trump Administration obstructs any advancements in the following progressive health policies that could benefit rural populations:

1. Social infrastructure: Government funding for programs to support the growing population of immigrants in rural communities could incentive spending and benefit the rural economy
2. Healthcare infrastructure – Rural hospitals profit from Medicaid expansion
3. Healthcare utilization – rural adults and children have greater access to healthcare facilities due to coverage from Medicaid/CHIP, thus avoiding health conditions that could lead to morbidity or premature death
4. Public health infrastructure – maintaining basic healthcare plans that require provisions for essential health benefits offers preventive screening measures to low income people

The trickle down effect, especially with the current Administration's tax reform intentions will only place rural Americans further behind, widening the income inequality gap and provoking greater geographical health disparities.

References

Altman, D. *How American feel about immigration and Muslims in a time of Donald Trump*, The Henry J. Kaiser Family Foundation. September 30, 2016. Retrieved from: https://www.kff.org/other/perspective/how-americans-feel-about-immigration-and-muslims-in-a-time-of-donald-trump/

American Civil Liberties Union. (2006). *Cracks in the system: Twenty years of the unjust crack cocaine law*. Retrieved from: https://www.aclu.org/files/assets/cracksinsystem_20061025.pdf

American College of Physicians. (March 6, 2017). *ACP says despite changes, revised immigration executive order will cause health care crises and encourage discrimination*. Retrieved from: https://www.acponline.org/acp-newsroom/acp-says-despite-changes-revised-immigration-executive-order-will-cause-health-care-crises-and

American Hospital Association. (2016). *CAH legislative history*. Retrieved from: http://www.aha.org/advocacy-issues/cah/history.shtml

Association for American Medical Colleges. (March 6, 2017). *AAMC statement on president Trump's revised executive order on immigration*. Retrieved from: https://news.aamc.org/press-releases/article/immigration_order_03062017/

Bernstein, J. *Jared Bernstein testimony: Tax expenditures: How cutting spending through the tax code can lower the deficit, improve efficiency, and boost fairness in the US tax code*. Center for Budget and Public Priorities. March 5, 2013. Retrieved from: https://www.cbpp.org/jared-bernstein-testimony-tax-expenditures-how-cutting-spending-through-the-tax-code-can-lower-the

Broaddus, M. *Affordable care Act's medicaid expansion benefits hospitals, particularly in Rural America*. June 23, 2017. Center for Budget and Public Priorities. Retrieved from: https://www.cbpp.org/research/health/affordable-care-acts-medicaid-expansion-benefits-hospitals-particularly-in-rural

Centers for Medicare and Medicaid Services. (2017a). *Rural community hospital demonstration program*. Retrieved from: https://innovation.cms.gov/initiatives/Rural-Community-Hospital/

Centers for Medicare and Medicaid Services. (2017b). *Fiscal Year (FY) 2018 medicare hospital Inpatient Prospective Payment System (IPPS) and Long Term Acute Care Hospital (LTCH) Prospective Payment System Final Rule (CMS-1677-F)*. Retrieved from: https://www.cms.gov/Newsroom/MediaReleaseDatabase/Fact-sheets/2017-Fact-Sheet-items/2017-08-02.html

Center for Rural Affairs. (May 30, 2017). *Immigration, opportunity and Rural America*. Retrieved from: https://www.cfra.org/news/170530/immigration-opportunity-and-rural-america

Committee on the Judiciary. (2017). *The sentencing reform and corrections Act of 2017*. Retrieved from: https://www.judiciary.senate.gov/imo/media/doc/Sentencing,%2010-04-17,%20SRCA%20115%20Summary.pdf

Davis, J. (2017). Health care reform is Just warming up. *Physician Leadership Journal, 4*(4), 10.

Díaz, J. J. (2011). Immigration policy, criminalization and the growth of the immigration industrial complex: Restriction, expulsion, and eradication of undocumented in the U.S. *Western Criminology Review, 12*(2), 35–54.

Evich, H. B. Revenge of the rural voter. *Politico*. November 13, 2016.

Foutz, J., Artiga, S., & Garfield, R. *The role of Medicaid in rural America*, The Henry J. Kaiser Family Foundation. April 25, 2017. Retrieved from: https://www.kff.org/medicaid/issue-brief/the-role-of-medicaid-in-rural-america/

Gale, W., & Krupkin, A. *Tax reform needed now!* The Brookings Institutions October 6, 2016. Retrieved from: https://www.brookings.edu/research/tax-reform-needed-now/

Hincks, J. (2017). CEOs from more than 400 leading U.S. companies urge trump to keep DACA. *Fortune.Com*, 26.

Howell, R. (2004). Sentencing reform lessons: From the sentencing reform act of 1984 to the Feeney amendment. *Journal of Criminal Law & Criminology, 94*(4), 1069–1104.

Huang, C., Herrera, G., & Brendan, D. *JCT estimates: Final GOP tax bill skewed to top, hurts many low- and middle-income Americans*. Center for Budget and Policy Priorities. December 19, 2017. Retrieved from: https://www.cbpp.org/research/federal-tax/jct-estimates-final-gop-tax-bill-skewed-to-top-hurts-many-low-and-middle-income

Institute on Taxation and Immigration Policy. (2017). State and local tax contributions of young undocumented immigrants. Retrieved from: https://itep.org/state-local-tax-contributions-of-young-undocumented-immigrants/#.WP9twPnytaS

Jan, T. White House claims 'dreamers' take jobs away from blacks and Hispanics. Here's the truth. *Washington Post*, September 6, 2017. https://www.washingtonpost.com/news/wonk/wp/2017/09/06/white-house-claims-dreamers-take-jobs-away-from-blacks-and-hispanics-heres-the-truth/?hpid=hp_rhp-more-top-stories_dacalawsuit-450pm:homepage/story&utm_term=.618a7256c8f5

Jessop, R. (2002). *The future of the capitalist state*. Blackwell publishing Inc., Malden MA.

Joint Economic Committee. (2017). *Rural DACA by the numbers*. Retrieved from: https://www.jec.senate.gov/public/_cache/files/e02f2015-ab3a-47aa-aa6f-215a1db74986/rural-daca-by-the-numbers.pdf

Kissam, E. *An evaluation of census 2010 coverage of rural hard-to-count tracts in California*. Proceedings of the 2012 conference on hard-to-count populations, American Statistical Association, December, 2012.

Leonard, R. Why rural America voted for trump. *The New York Times*. January 5, 2017.

Luthra, S. (2017). Unhealthy Delusions. *Newsweek Global, 167*(26), 50–51.

Manuel, C. P. (2017). Of cultural backlash and economic insecurity in the 2016 American presidential election. *Política & Sociedade: Revista De Sociologia Política, 16*(36), 212–227.

McGraw, M., Kelsey, A., & Keneally, M. A timeline of Trump's immigration executive order and legal challenges. *ABC News,* June 29, 2017.

Minier, J. (2017). *Immigrants benefit the community and economy*. Lexington: University of Kentucky Center for Equality and Social Justice.

Mueller, K., Coburn, A., Lundblad, J., MacKinney, A., McBride, T., & Watson, S. (2012). *The current and future role and impact of medicaid in rural health*. Retrieved from: http://www.rupri.org/Forms/HealthPanel_Medicaid:Sept2012.pdf

National Conference of State Legislators. (2017). *Closing the gaps in the rural primary care workforce*. Retrieved from: http://www.ncsl.org/research/health/closing-the-gaps-in-the-rural-primary-care-workfor.aspx

National Immigration Law Center. (2009). Facts about internal revenue service no-match letters. Retrieved from: https://www.nilc.org/issues/workersrights/irs-nomatch/

Newman, E. (2017). DACA's fate worries healthcare industry. *Mcknight's Long-Term Care News, 38*(10), 1.

O'Hare, W. (2007). *Rural children increasingly rely on medicaid and SCHIP*. Carsey Institute. Retrieved from: http://www.borderhealth.org/files/res_886.pdf

Parmet, W. E., Sainsbury-Wong, L., & Prabhu, M. (2017). Immigration and health: Law, policy, and ethics. *Journal of Law, Medicine & Ethics, 45*, 55–59.

Quinn, M. Spending deal offers short-term CHIP relief. *Governing the States and Localities*. December 11, 2017.

Richardson, D. Trump administration expands prison-industrial complex for deportations. *Observer,* October 18, 2017.

Stone, C. *Ending DACA program for young undocumented immigrants makes no economic sense*, Center for Budget and Public Priorities. September 27, 2017. Retrieved from: https://www.cbpp.org/research/economy/ending-daca-program-for-young-undocumented-immigrants-makes-no-economic-sense#_ftn5

Surowiecki, J. (2016). Trump sets private prisons free. *New Yorker, 92*(40), 26.

The Henry J. Kaiser Family Foundation. (2017a). *Kaiser Family Foundation/Washington post partnership survey probes experiences and views of Rural Americans*. June 19, 2017. Retrieved from: https://www.kff.org/health-reform/press-release/kaiser-family-foundationwashington-post-partnership-survey-probes-experiences-and-views-of-rural-americans/

The Henry J. Kaiser Family Foundation. (2017b). *Key facts about the uninsured population*. Retrieved from: http://www.kff.org/uninsured/fact-sheet/key-facts-about-the-uninsured-population

The Henry J. Kaiser Family Foundation. (2017c). *The affordable care act and insurance coverage in rural areas*. Retrieved from: http://www.kff.org/uninsured/issue-brief/the-affordable-care-act-and-insurance-coverage-in-rural-areas/

The Henry J. Kaiser Family Foundation. (2017d). *Changes in insurance coverage in rural areas under the ACA: A focus on medicaid expansion states*. May 4, 2017. Retrieved from: https://www.kff.org/medicaid/fact-sheet/changes-in-insurance-coverage-in-rural-areas-under-the-aca-a-focus-on-medicaid-expansion-states/

The Henry J. Kaiser Family Foundation. (2017e). *Interactive maps: Estimates of enrollment in ACA marketplaces and medicaid expansion*. October 4, 2017. Retrieved from: https://www.kff.org/interactive/interactive-maps-estimates-of-enrollment-in-aca-marketplaces-and-medicaid-expansion/

The Henry J. Kaiser Family Foundation. (2017f). *Next steps for CHIP: What is at stake for children?* June 13, 2017. Retrieved from: https://www.kff.org/medicaid/fact-sheet/next-steps-for-chip-what-is-at-stake-for-children/

The Henry J. Kaiser Family Foundation. (2017g). *State plans for CHIP as federal CHIP funds run out*. December 6, 2017. Retrieved from: https://www.kff.org/medicaid/fact-sheet/state-plans-for-chip-as-federal-chip-funds-run-out

The Henry J. Kaiser Family Foundation. *Legislative summary: State children's health insurance program – Fact Sheet*. November 29, 1997. Retrieved from: https://www.kff.org/medicaid/fact-sheet/legislative-summary-state-childrens-health-insurance-program-2/

Toder, E., & Viard, A. *Major surgery needed: A call for structural reform of the U.S. Corporate Income Tax*. Tax Policy Center, Urban Institute and Brookings Institution. April 3, 2014. Retrieved from: http://www.taxpolicycenter.org/publications/major-surgery-needed-call-structural-reform-us-corporate-income-tax

U.S. Citizenship and Immigration Services. (2017). *E-Verify*. Retrieved from: https://www.uscis.gov/e-verify

U.S. Department of Justice. *Attorney general sessions delivers remarks on DACA*. U.S. Department of Justice, September 5, 2017., https://www.justice.gov/opa/speech/attorney-general-sessions-delivers-remarks-daca

Washington State Sentencing Guidelines Commission. (2017). *Sentencing reform Act: Historical background*. Retrieved from: http://ofm.wa.gov/sgc/documents/historical.pdf

Willison, C. E., & Singer, P. M. (2017). Repealing the affordable care act essential health benefits: Threats and obstacles. *American Journal of Public Health, 107*(8), 1225–1226.

Chapter 5
Conclusion: Political Economy: An Era of Institutional Cynicism?

One salient theme prevails throughout this book – that is, economic theory drives political choices, which in turn, determines social conditions. If neoliberal ideology is the economic order of interest, then tension for resources and subsequently social disorder becomes more prevalent.

Capitalist profit from social disorder through political decision-making to invest less in public welfare programs and ambitious legislation to accelerate incarceration rates. Prison expansion occurred when the data did not demonstrate a demand for additional prison beds. Policymakers passed legislation that posed harsher penalties for crimes ubiquitous to the poor. It is no surprise that poorer people are concentrated in U.S. prisons. Also, not surprisingly, more of the rural poor are occupying the prisons.

Marxist theory on the political economy holds some relevance to the discourse on rural health disparities. Marxist theory implicated economic ideologies rooted in capital accumulation, compromised political behaviors and ultimately caused social unrest. The prison industrial complex led to massive arrests of African American men with long term mandatory sentences for nonviolent drug crimes. Conspiracy theories and social movements emerged in opposition, calling for criminal justice reform. Racial profiling resulted in low income blacks and minorities sharing the burden of arrests, which sparked class and racial tensions. Similarily, the immigration industrial complex and the passage of Federal legislation, provoked additional policing and more recently, immigrant profiling. The end of DACA will further complicate social disorder and economic instability, stimulating social unrest, including from the Fortune 500 companies that employ DACA participants. The criminal justice system has not been reformed in nearly 50 years. In the absence of reform, the prison industry continues to profit substantially.

Marxists theory prevails on the economic causes for rural health disparities. Marx saw class struggle as a result of a neoliberal social order. Historically, rural populations experienced higher prevalence of poverty, were less educated and employment opportunities were insufficient. If policymakers considered equalizing

© The Author(s) 2018   47
M. M. Taylor, *Application of the Political Economy to Rural Health Disparities*,
SpringerBriefs in Public Health, https://doi.org/10.1007/978-3-319-73537-5_5

the distribution of income, this would force states to address policies germane to resource allocation. For example, why are job growth or job opportunities unequally distributed across geographical lines? Policies fostering job growth through incentives to Corporations could alleviate the employment challenges in this region. Raising the minimum wage to meet the real cost of living in states can narrow income inequality levels. Also, boosting the farming industry is plausible and could revive productivity in rural locales. However, farmers can not compete with Agri-Businesses, and without government intervention on behalf of farmers, the concepts in the political economy of geography prevails!

Political decisions to invest – not only in the actual budget for education, but in programs that foster educational attainment in primary and secondary schools in rural areas would offer young adults options for economic mobility. This could alleviate the disproportionate levels of pregnancy among rural teens. Single female headed households, which account for a large share of high poverty rates in rural areas, can be reduced. Consequently, child poverty rates would decrease, avoiding stagnated intergenerational mobility.

Retrenchment of public welfare programs benefit Corporations and wealthy Americans. The current Administration's tax reform bill substantiates this reality. Threats to repeal the provisions in the ACA will only result in greater rural health disparities. Preventive health care for rural populations would be even more out of their reach. Excess morbidity in chronic and infectious diseases and a lack of program investments for substance abuse disorders only leads to loss of productivity, morbidity or worse, premature deaths among rural populations. Expanding health care options would only benefit rural populations. Consequently, healthcare capitalists stand to profit more if rural health disparities worsen.

The political economy approach, is indeed, applicable to rural health disparities. The lack of economic commitment from government to improve access to goods and services for rural communities compromises their health and wealth being. Market justice and wealth accumulation is visibly fundamental to the current political doctrine. But, fairness in the geographical redistribution of critical resources appears to be common sense – unless, however, we are living in the political economy era of institutional cynicism?

Index

© The Author(s) 2018   49
M. M. Taylor, *Application of the Political Economy to Rural Health Disparities*,
SpringerBriefs in Public Health, https://doi.org/10.1007/978-3-319-73537-5

Printed in the United States
By Bookmasters